HUMANS BEING

Creating Your Life From the Inside Out

LOU ANN DALY, PH.D.

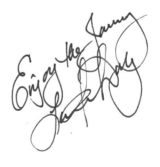

AuthorHouse™
1663 Liberty Drive
Bloomington, IN 47403
www.authorhouse.com
Phone: 1-800-839-8640

First published by AuthorHouse 6/11/2009

ISBN: 978-1-4389-6596-3 (sc)

Library of Congress Control Number: 2009903107

Printed in the United States of America
Bloomington, Indiana

This book is printed on acid-free paper.

authorHOUSE®

Dedication

This book is dedicated with much gratitude to:

Mom, Dad, and Aunt Jean, who have always supported my journey in every way they could, even as they are still trying to figure out what I do for a living,

Fred Miller who journeys on wings wherever he goes, and

most especially my dear friend and colleague Lynn Potoff without whose encouragement, guidance, and support, this book would at best be unreadable and at worst sitting in my computer for several more years.

Acknowledgments

To the dear friends and tireless editors of so many versions of this manuscript I thank you for your advice, wisdom, and commitment to this work and its potential in this world. In particular, I want to acknowledge the help of readers and editors Bea Mah Holland, Cheryl Taustin, Marcie Anthone , Kellie Wardman, Diane Fritschle, Ann Wright, Pat Zalewski, and Lynn Potoff who read—and reread this book many times. Thank you for your patience, your encouragement, and your unwavering support.

To my contributors Lula and Thembi, thank you for so generously sharing your time and stories with me and the many readers who will benefit from your voice and experience. Thank you also to Sydney Bevins for artistically handling the technological aspects of my illustrations.

To the many O! LAD workshop participants around the world who have been engaging their own journeys and touching my life and the lives of others with their insights, thank you for testing and validating the concepts and exercises in this book over the years.

To the women in my Wise Women's Circle—Bea, Kathleen, Marg, and Kellie—thank you for encouraging and prodding me every step of the way, while also tapping into every connection you could think of to get this book to press.

And finally, to all who have shared in any aspect of enabling this book to see the light of day, I offer my gratitude. Your gift is not only to me but also to all who use its contents to realize their potential and gifts.

Many thanks.

Table of Contents

Imagine the Impact

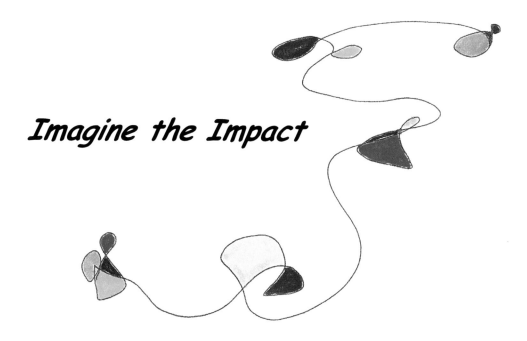

If one cell can mutate and multiply to the point of transforming a healthy body, imagine what one healthy person who touches and inspires others can do. Imagine a world filled with people who choose joy, health, and peace, people who foster abundance rather than scarcity. What if I told you this is not a pipe dream if you choose to make it real? Stop for a moment and think about how your impact on the health of the world could transform lives today if you choose to lead life from your heart. Imagine.

What would be possible in places of learning around the world?

With more conscious teachers, staff, and administrators, schools could become cultures of celebration where diversity is welcomed, embraced, and sought for the richness it brings to the learning experience. Students would learn from role models how to live from the wisdom of their hearts and greet differences with receptivity and curiosity. Differences would become growth opportunities rather than sources of fear and alienation.

When administrators see their work as creating environments where all school personnel celebrate contributions—in whatever form they take—there will be a place for everyone to bring whatever gifts she or he has. Our educational systems would change—one teacher, one administrator, one custodian at a time. By building on a foundation of leaders "being," becoming more whole as individuals, and creating cultures of celebration, teachers and other school leaders would create a whole new context for learning, and a brighter future for learners.

What could happen if social systems change?

Imagine what would be possible when the leaders and workers focus less on heroic rescuing and more on helping those they serve to live into their own gifts and potential. Imagine what could change when the leaders choose to reconnect with their hearts and disconnect from ego-driven roles where they unconsciously take accountability for other people's lives. By unconsciously doing what we have always done in large social systems such as health care and child and family services, we create cultures of entitlement, dependency, and hopelessness. These are not the qualities that result from conscious choice and courage.

What is possible when people see others in need and consciously choose to help is what happens whenever we experience a natural disaster. People step into the Highest in themselves and focus on raising others up, until those in need can help themselves. What if our social systems did the same? Imagine what could happen if social systems were designed to remind people that their voices make a difference and their gifts matter. No more focus on hand outs; instead hands would be outstretched contributing and sharing the abundance of gifts in all people.

What could happen if business leaders drive conscious choices in the workplace?

Imagine what it would be like for leaders at every level of an organization to consciously consider who they will be, what they will stand for, and what kinds of organizational cultures they will make their personal legacy.

Conversations would change to support courageous decision-making, rather than fear-based silence or withdrawal. Intentions would matter. The ways we treat each other in getting the work done would matter. We could learn to see the whole person instead of the role someone holds in the organization. Imagine what it could be like to work in a company that inspires its people to develop themselves and each other, rather than fear and compete with each other.

It would not be so difficult to imagine a workplace where the whole person comes to work and people communicate in ways that continuously support the best in themselves and in each other. Imagine working in such workplaces everyday—and imagine the levels of inspired innovation and business results!

How could being more conscious change parenting?

Imagine remembering—in every interaction—the dreams you hold for your child and for the kind of parent you want to be with him or her.

Conscious parents would return to the clarity of their heart to ask whether the way they are behaving or choosing to respond in a particular situation is consistent with the kind of parent they choose to be. Conscious parents would be acutely aware of their own gifts and passions, modeling for their children the journey of following their hearts.

Imagine how our children would be raised when parents feel celebrated, valued, and connected with what is Highest in them. Imagine.

If we were more conscious, what kind of world could we create?

What does it take to create a world where people live into their potential while supporting the best in each other? It takes conscious choice—that's it. By waking up to what our hearts know and choosing to follow the wisdom and truth of our very being, we create a place for individuals, communities, and whole nations to prosper.

World peace starts with inner peace and inner peace starts with going inward to discern what is true in your heart. The awareness that comes from living that truth creates a spirit of generosity, grace, and gratitude. It is about listening, not telling. It is about asking who people want to be and what they want to create. It is about raising each other up to fulfill dreams. It is not about who gets more. Awareness means knowing that there is enough for everyone.

More conscious people would experience inner peace and create environments where others learn that they can have the same, if they choose. Leaders would live into their potential. Abundance. Clarity. Courage. This is leadership from the inside out. It is about being. The conscious path for each person relies on connecting with the wisdom and truth inside. And the good news is that everyone can have access. Inner peace. World peace. The invitation is open to everyone—to you. You choose.

Imagine the impact.

I see it every day in the people who make the choice to discover the truth in their hearts. These people come from different geographies, communities, social classes, ethnicities, genders, and ages. They come from all walks of life. What they have in common is the willingness and desire to discover how to make a difference by being different, by choosing to follow their truth, and by helping others to do the same.

These wonderful people are working at high levels in business and education and on the front lines in all kinds of companies and organizations. They are parents and children, friends, and managers. Some are preparing to retire, others to start families of their own. All inspire others by their courage to stand tall when conventional wisdom and outside forces don't support their decisions. And all teach by being, by sharing the dream, and having the courage to live from their hearts.

They are learning to listen to the wisdom of their hearts. And they are learning to trust their own wisdom over the norms of social convention and rules for belonging that curb their uniqueness and individuality. They are exploring how to stay true to themselves while creating more opportunities for friends and co-workers to be true to the best in themselves. They are learning to stay present—to pay attention to what is happening and to what they feel in each moment. They are reconnecting with the joy of following their passions and rediscovering what those passions are.

They are paying attention to how they distract themselves from being present every day by listening to the voices in their heads that remind them what they "should" be doing. And they are learning to let go and dance with life's playful rhythms. Just as important, they are developing networks of support to help each other find their Highest potential, step into it, and relish every moment of discovery. They are stepping with more confidence into the full power of their individual and collective voices—something we desperately need in our world today.

We are living in a time of massive institutional failure. Our large social systems—government, economy, education, health care, business, religion, social services, and others—have been imploding under the weight of blind conformity to structures that have long since outlived their intended purpose. As we become more conscious and more awake, individuals are speaking up more about what is called for in this period in our history. We hear more about the need for a new world order. It is a simpler, more inclusive order that calls us to be accountable for leading our own lives and choosing how to invest our energy. It can't come from the old ways of thinking—that being complicated and difficult makes something more important, or that some outside authority will provide the answers.

We need exactly the opposite. It is time to start from simple truths. It is time to look inward for answers—not outward to authority figures and media to give events meaning. It is time to accept nothing without asking if it is true for your heart today. Know your own wisdom and truth, and shine your light for others to do the same—in their own time and in their own ways.

This book is about that journey inward to the heart and conscious choice. It is about the world we can create together when we choose consciously from the heart and help each other to keep doing so every day. The choice is yours. It is always yours.

Imagine the life you want to lead and the impact you want to have.

You choose.

The Journey

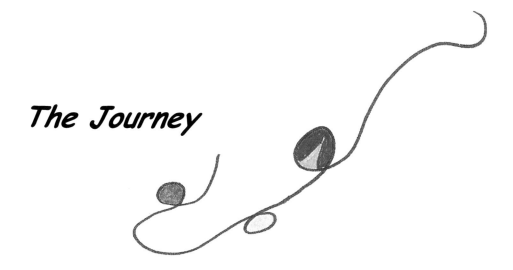

Did you know there is a whole conspiracy of support for you having a life of meaning, ease, and joy? Not feeling it? Check again. It is there. Are you aware of how much energy you use fighting the path of ease and personal fulfillment? Seriously, your life and everything in it either leads you to walk your own path with sheer delight and lightness or to unconsciously impose challenges and burdens that distract you from your own calling. In the latter case, your choices at best provide moments of respite, at worst continuous pain.

The life of joy, profound peace, and fulfillment is a life lived consciously. Stop for a moment and reflect on that. What that statement means is that for you to have the life of your dreams, you need to be awake—and keep your eyes wide open throughout. It does not have to be scary. It does not have to be dark or heavy. In fact, it can be simply delightful, engaging, and wondrous—if that is what you choose. Here is how it works:

Each choice to be true to your Highest Self leads closer to a life of purpose; each distraction from living your truth takes you away. You experience fulfillment and meaningfulness when you stand in your own light and operate from truth, instead of living in the shadow of your potential. Remember that your purpose is yours. No one else can access the truth of your heart as you can. The essence of who you become when you feel joyful, when you feel light and free, when you are able to see the gifts in all that happens is your Highest Self. We all have one. It is our truth. Sometimes it gets buried under everyday distractions, but it is there—always.

If you consider that you are perfectly designed at the core to lead a life of experiences that serve the highest and best in you, you begin to look at your health, qualities, gifts, and dreams differently. The package you arrived in—your physical body—serves your purpose. Do you know how? Are you using it effectively? The unique gifts and talents that make you who you are support your purpose. Do you know how? Are you using them in a way that feels true and uplifting to you or are you trying to conform to others' expectations of you?

What makes your life one of ease and joy is how you choose to respond to whatever happens and who-ever walks into or out of your life. Fundamentally and most simply, your heart knows your purpose; and your head—which is filled with the voices of others that you have internalized over the years (all the shoulds and ought to's)—presents inviting ways to distract you from your path, choosing instead to stay in the perceived comfort of the status quo. In the distracted life, you lead with your head; in the conscious life, you lead with your heart. You need both head and heart. Which one leads makes all the difference.

That's it. That's really all there is. The rest is about "how". So for those of you who like ideas and think you already "got it," you may not want to read the rest of this book. For those of you who want to do something that can reconnect you with your light, laughter, and truth, the rest of the book is designed to help you on the path. Get cozy. The journey is quite enjoyable, if you give yourself permission to relax.

One of the first things you may encounter is the realization that you have lost touch with who you are. Many people do not have any real idea of *who they are*, what brings them joy, what fills them with mean-ing, excitement, and profound peace. Instead, they define themselves and their lives by *what they do*, the hats they wear, and the titles or roles they fill. Any identity of Self with "doing" is a distraction that takes you off path.

WHO YOU ARE ≠ WHAT YOU DO

If what you do brings you joy and fills you with energy, keep doing it. If not, stop it. The choice is yours to stay or change. Distract yourself from your heart's desires or wake up and choose who you will be and what brings you joy.

The path to conscious living, eyes wide open, does not need to be dark or difficult. In fact, I know it to be irresistibly funny, an adventure of the highest making, and open to everyone who chooses it. So pre-pare to let go of self-criticism and guilt. There is no room for these two responses to life here. Drama doesn't fit either. If your identity is built on melodrama and you are not willing to let go of that drama, you are probably not ready for this particular approach. Nothing personal. It just won't work for you.

This journey is about reconnecting with your brilliant and most engaging Self. It is about discovering or re-discovering the things that most tickle you and then choosing how to design your life with them in it. It is about understanding a few fundamentals that support all of us on earth in living consciously. And it is about cultivating the soil in which to plant and grow your Highest Self in every context in which you find yourself.

As with the process of life itself, it is not complicated. It is elegantly simple. Life is not difficult. Hu-mans who are not awake make it so, but Life itself isn't. The entire process can be described on a simple little organic grid that is defined by two core processes and two points of contact.

The grid is called the Universal Soul Grid, because it applies to all conscious life forms (that would be you and me for starters). It works like this:

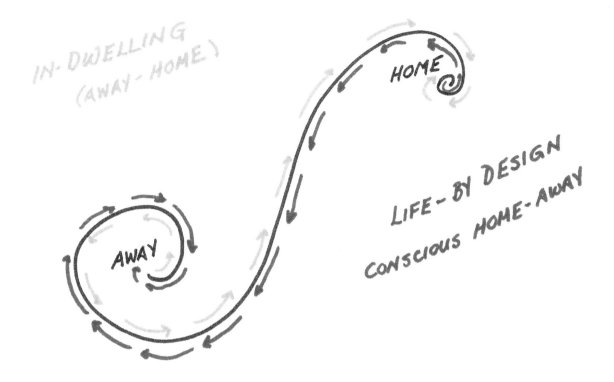

First there is a contact point called *Home*. Home refers to who you are when you are your Highest Self. It holds your truth and wisdom. It is the best and highest in you, prior to any "lessons" learned in life. It is your inner world. *Away* is the only other contact point and it refers to the world of human standards, rules for success, and social conventions about what is considered right and wrong, good and bad, success and failure. It refers to your outer or external world.

The two processes that support conscious living are:

    • the shift from unconscious relationship with external forces and head distractions to conscious relationship with your heart, Truth, and Highest Self –the path from Away towards Home, and

    • the conscious integration of the inner world of Highest Self with the outer world of human relationships and everyday life—the path from Home to Away

The first process is called In-Dwelling. It is the journey inward to reconnect with your deepest passions and wisdom. The second process is called Conscious Living or Living—By Design. This process is the one that helps you to change your relationships with every part of your life in ways that support the Best and Highest in you and the people you touch.

Go inward to rekindle your relationship with your Highest Self,

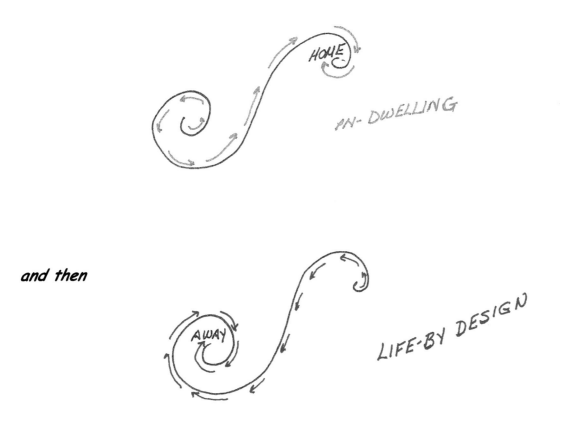

and then

bring your truth and greatest contributions to the external world to create a different kind of global community than the one we are living in today.

What makes each of our lives so different and unique is how we engage these two processes. The path to stepping into your gifts and living your dreams more consciously can be easily mapped on the Universal Soul Grid, as can the path to distraction, drama, and pain.

Humans Being offers you tips to more consciously navigate the path of the Soul Grid through the transitions in your life, to reconnect with your Self, your truths, your passions, and your deepest desires, and to take that magnificent Self into all aspects of your life. Humans Being will also guide you in living into your gifts in ways that keep your eyes wide open to distractions that could cause pain and struggle so that you can change the patterns in your life. You will find that as you choose what you love, you will naturally create the space and opportunity for others—family, friends, colleagues, and even strangers—to do the same. Rather than viewing others as competition, you begin to inspire the best in your Self and others by bringing the best of your Self to every relationship and situation.

This book offers stories and tips from others' journeys as well as exercises to help you on your path. Use them as they serve you. The path along the Soul Grid will be charted, along with opportunities for you to discover where you hold yourself back (most often unconsciously) from magnificence and sheer joy. You listened to the voice that keeps telling you there is more. Trust it again. The only step that awaits you is the next one on your path. Take it. It matters. It really matters. You already know this. That's why you're here.

In Service of Truth...and Ease

There are some things that are true about the way life happens, whether we choose to recognize them or not. Denying them or distracting ourselves from dealing with them will not make them less true and will not make them disappear. The first and most basic is that all living things are constantly changing and growing. They do so in ways that either produce or erode their continued health and ability to flourish.

We humans are the only species—that I know of, anyway—that puts change out there as something to be feared, managed, and controlled. At some level it's time to get real. Every cell in our body is alive and changing all the time. Because we can't see change happening, we may dismiss it as irrelevant or not worthy of our attention. Every seven years or so, we will have regenerated the cells in our bodies. That is significant change! In the same way, we age a little bit everyday, but somehow seem shocked at how we reached thirty, forty, fifty, sixty, seventy, or eighty years of age and are wherever we find ourselves at those points. It is as if life happened to us and then we are surprised with what it brought.

We tend to pay attention to and give meaning to changes that disrupt whatever path we are on or thought we were on. Then we stop to notice. For example, you may love your job for several days, weeks, months, or years and then realize at some point that it is not fulfilling, or just simply doesn't work for you anymore. This "sudden" awareness of what is happening can apply to marriages, partnerships, your relationship with your Self, your work, your beliefs, and with other situations in which you find yourself.

If you stop to examine what is going on, you recognize that you have been less than satisfied for a while. Rather than acknowledge the initial inklings that something was not serving to bring out the best in you, you listened to one of those voices in your head that distracted you from doing something to change the situation. Maybe it's the voice that directs you to be happy with what you have, that now is not the time to change anything, or the one that says it will only be the same if you go anywhere else, so just learn to accept where you are and deal with it. Whatever you told yourself to shut down the awareness that something was not serving your Best Self, it was a mind distraction from the truth in your heart.

Typically, what we do is to keep upping the ante with more and more self talk, or we choose some other way to numb the awareness of the heart's message by self-medicating—compulsively rewarding ourselves with food, new toys or other indulgences for putting up with less than exhilarating lives. These tactics or medications can take forms like the obviously unproductive ones of soothing ourselves with comfort foods, alcohol, or other drugs of choice to the less obvious distractions of staying busy and focusing on being "productive". Compulsive anything, whether shopping or exercising, can serve to numb or distract us from paying attention to the body signals and emotions trying to get our attention that we are not feeling fulfilled, not acting on our own wisdom, and that we are off path.

The beauty of these wonderful signals that we work so hard to deny, shut down, and otherwise dismiss is that they are all part of a conspiracy to help us choose purposeful lives, to help us live into our potential—strongly, boldly, and with vibrancy. We are using our energy in life to distract ourselves from seeing, feeling, hearing, or otherwise acknowledging these signals. Why? So that we don't have to change whatever is causing us to be off track, less than satisfied, or feeling empty? The logic of this behavior would be…?

Change is natural. It is occurring all the time. It carries no meaning. It is neither good nor bad. Only in the context of what we *think* we want our lives to be and how we *expect* life to happen, does change become a challenge.

> *Life is happening—whether we like it or not!*
> *It just is. That's all.*
> *No hidden meaning. No deep message. Life happens.*
> *What really matters is how we respond.*

Life goes on whether we pay attention to it or not. At some point, all that has been happening suddenly hits a critical point where we wake up and pay attention. Usually these points are points of frustration or anger, sometimes illness or pure exhaustion, often because the world did not respond as we had expected or planned. Our way of being has been disturbed in a way that gets our attention. Maybe the promotion you were expecting did not happen. Maybe you are ready to admit that the career in which you find yourself is draining your energy and creativity. At this critical point, you are invited to really see what is happening and choose to change something to make your life easier and truer to the person you want to be. This course of action means letting go of how you wanted, expected, or planned for your life to unfold.

Unfortunately, the alternative path is the one more often taken. This path is where you choose to use your willpower and energy to override or deny what you experience and resist whatever is happening. You escape into your head and re-focus on what you convince yourself "should" be happening. You tell yourself to be thankful that you have a job, even one that drains your energy. Rather than seizing the opportunity to examine whether the path you are on is really working for you, you find yourself instead lamenting what is happening and declaring it to be unfair—after all, you don't deserve this! You judge the system that gave someone else a promotion to be biased. You muster the willpower and emotions to fight the way things are unfolding, and then use even more energy to resist.

Given the opportunity to live with our eyes wide open, see what is unfolding, look life squarely in the eye and determine how to respond in a way that reminds us to reach higher and enjoy who we are, we choose to live out the drama in our heads about the "way it's supposed to be." No wonder we feel stressed!

Any form of resistance creates stress. Consider this whenever you are looking at whether your life is free, fulfilling, and meaningful, or burdened and heavy. What are you resisting that is actually there to serve you by disrupting your current choices and inviting you to open your eyes wide to how you feel, who you are becoming, and what the wisdom of your heart is telling you? You are invited to recognize the conspiracy of benign forces supporting your highest potential. The more you resist, the more you will be shown opportunities to consider where you are denying your own brilliance and joy.

Two illustrations of life happening, distractions taking hold, and individual awakenings appear in the following stories. The first is about a woman we'll call Lila.

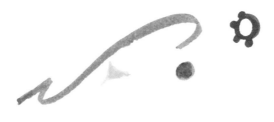

LILA'S STORY

A wildly imaginative child, Lila began to see herself as a misfit as early as kindergarten. In her family she felt accepted by one parent but not understood. She was a sensitive child who learned to retreat into her own realm for sanity and solace. Her retreat inward was accelerated at age twelve when her parents divorced. She became the parent to her siblings when her parents were unable to fill the role. Lila's whimsical nature and wild imaginings no longer fit with the new role of responsible adult. She retreated further inward.

She carried feelings of being a misfit into adulthood and with her through several corporate positions. Retreating to creative ways to survive the unwelcome grasp of corporate conformity, she often helped others who felt like misfits and outcasts to feel good about themselves and their contributions. Extremely successful at getting things done in a harsh and somewhat convoluted system of big egos, she skillfully protected staff, encouraged their personal development, and limited her own. When the emotional and physical cost of staying in such an ill-fitting environment for her became too high, physical symptoms pushed her to face her own fears about leaving.

A step in the decision to leave the debilitating corporate environment was to address the insecurity of being financially dependent on another person. Having seen the negative impact of financial dependence of one parent on the other when her parents divorced Lila did not want to create the same situation in her life. She and her husband developed a financial plan for her to be able to leave the toxic work situation. Together they worked to get their house in order. She needed to figure out for herself how much financial dependency she would allow herself in order to create the freedom to heal and explore her inner Self.

When Lila began to think about her exit from business, she had some vague awareness about expressing her creativity, but was much clearer about what she did not want than what she did want. She really did not know what would make her happiest, but she had an idea or two, and knew the general parameters she wanted to test for herself. She and her husband worked on how they would scale back to support her leaving the corporate environment. Once she shifted her focus to pursuing her creativity, she was more prepared to take the leap. A few years after leaving her corporate position, Lila was firmly reconnected with her whimsical nature. She reported,

> *I like how I feel when I'm in my Highest Self. My own state of grace is magical.*

Having divorced herself from the large corporate system, she has been working through a debilitating auto-immune disease that continuously reminds her where she is spending her energy and whether she is nourishing her wonderfully whimsical nature and delightfully creative—and very competent—Self. She is painfully aware of both the power she gave to her corporate higher ups to validate her worth and the cost to her emotional and physical health of doing so.

As she shifted her energy and efforts to more creative enterprises that nourish her magical Self, she began to attract adults who sought her help in rediscovering their creative side. She became a leader in school activities that develop and nurture children's creative expression. Her lightness and playfulness are inspiring to her children and family. She is experimenting with work that is more satisfying and creative, while being aware of the wily voices that distract her from that creativity.

Lila has redefined what "responsible choices" look like, as well as how she wants to respond to her earlier desire to fit in with corporate and broader social expectations for success. She is now more attuned to people and projects that bring out, rather than deny, her magical Self. She withdraws from relationships that require her to be less than she is at her core. Today she continues to explore what work fits her unique gifts and Highest Self. Lila is more aware of the distractions she entertains in her life—and of the ultimate cost to her health. She is also quick to declare how much more alive she feels, having listened—finally—to the signals supporting her path. Her finances have not turned out to be the problem she had feared. Her relationships are healthier. Her pace has shifted. And she continues to pay attention to places where she can slip into being less than her heart knows she can be.

Another perspective comes from a woman whose life experiences appear to be very different, although you may recognize the similarities underlying distractions and choices made by the woman we'll call Estelle.

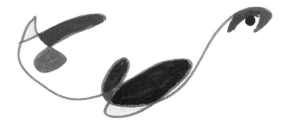

ESTELLE'S STORY

This woman was raised in a different era, with norms for race figuring very prominently in her journey to determine what "fitting in" would mean in her life.

When I was growing up, Black kids didn't have the options or role models to prepare us for college. For example, in elementary school, counselors and teachers guided Black kids, especially low income ones, into trades. There was no talk about going to college. And I knew I didn't want any of the trades.

In fourth and fifth grade, there was an African American school psychologist who was the first to graduate from our local university. She was showing herself as a role model. I didn't want any of the roles available to Black women at the time—teacher or social worker, so I decided to be a psychologist. Hell, I didn't even know what a psychologist was or did.

Having no plans to follow the path laid out in school for her, this woman went on to a series of successful careers, rising to senior positions naturally. She was told early on that there was something about the way she walked and carried her Self that was different from others. Her sense of Self was evident to others, even if she was not so consciously aware herself.

Her bent for questioning anything that didn't ring true or make rational sense guided her along a path that was not well worn in her own family. She constantly wrestled with fit. In the early days, she tried to fit in her family "just because" they were family. She would get dinners together and organize family events—only to find that invited family members couldn't get along with each other. Once she saw the pattern, she consciously decided that she would no longer support it. She dispensed with serving as peacemaker or primary caretaker and was not swayed by family members' attempts to reengage her in those efforts. Her clarity about how she would spend her energy and what relationships she would support allowed her to choose and act on what kind of fit with family she wanted to have.

Another area in which she sought "fit" was at Church. She grew up deeply entrenched in a fundamentalist church where the members of her family were significant leaders and where she, as a child, had "her place." She describes listening to the messages she heard in church about the way chosen people, good people, behaved and how only the people in church would be saved. She carefully surveyed the people in church and decided that she:

saw people drawing the box around themselves—"One way to God." And I looked around and saw whole lotta people in this world not in this room.

She literally thought about other people who were not in the room—people who were nice to her. They were excluded from the list of people who would make it to God and they seemed fine to her! So she concluded, "This is nuts." Estelle applied logic and reasoning based on her own experience, and detached from situations that made no sense by testing what she was being told against her actual experience. She developed a process of going inside herself to decide whether what she was hearing fit with the truth of her own experience.

Along the way, Estelle looked for data to discern and follow her path. She chose to step outside her family. At nineteen, she studied Eastern philosophies. It was the 1960's. Her boyfriend and friends affirmed her. There she would find a fit. She was a midwife in Chicago. She saw herself as a "nonconformist among non-conformists." She concluded that, "It must be God" that took her back to counting on her Self, based on what was true for her, even if it didn't match others' views. She never lost her abiding faith in God's place in her life, but she would not accept a relationship on earth or with God that didn't ring true for her. Estelle has been walking the path of testing fit her whole life. She pushes her own boundaries, questions her assumptions and beliefs, and works to discern her own truth.

The process of listening to those vague inklings, points of discomfort and dis-ease is the process of waking up to your truth and knowing who you are at your Center. It is a process of recognizing and naming distractions to which you give your power—for whatever human standard of success and validation. This is not the journey of a lone soul. While the individual stories vary in detail and texture, a core story begins to emerge. The story reveals a path of:

• Acquiring a social identity and losing our essential Selves

• Reaching points of awareness that where we are, who we have become, or who we are with is no longer fulfilling

• More consciously facing and addressing those relationships, qualities, beliefs, and things that don't fit us any longer

• Learning to make choices that support the full expression of our Best Selves, which in turn serve not only our unique potential but also the collective potential of the broader community

Not all of us have been engaging all aspects of this path. But its influence and prompting in your life become clear when you look squarely at who you are becoming, the results of your choices, and the relative ease or difficulty of your life. The simple truth in your heart—in whatever form you recognize it—serves your own unique journey. As long as you remember that point, faith and courage more easily follow. The desire to open your eyes and see where you invest your energy to hold yourself back—for whatever reason—becomes a curiosity, rather than a failure. And the possibility of greatness and living your dreams emerges much more clearly.

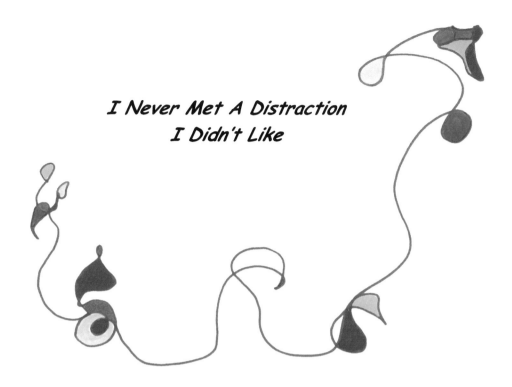

I Never Met A Distraction
I Didn't Like

On the journey to reconnect with who you are when you are your very Best or Highest Self, you are presented continuous opportunities to either become more conscious of your heart's passion, truth, and wisdom, or to distract yourself from ever getting there. These distractions will take various forms and will be reinforced by voices in your head. It may help you to think of these voices as "mind chatter" or noise on your path. When you unconsciously allow these voices to occupy the power position in your life, it's a little like owning a spectacular beach house and allowing whoever wants to live in it rent-free to do so. I don't know about you, but I want to enjoy that beach house with whomever I select to be there with me. If you feel the same way, it is time to open your eyes and wander into the theatre in your head to see what distraction is playing that takes you away from being alive and present in every moment of your life.

Remember to lighten up! It is time to get a kick out of what you see and who you meet. Resist the temptation to judge where you are, who you have become, and what choices you have made. How you spend your time may have you shaking your head—do so with lightness and humor. Your heart and soul know truth, not judgments. Judgments are not going to serve you on this part of the journey. It doesn't matter if you are reading this at the age of eighty, eighteen, forty-eight, or fifty-four. It doesn't matter how long you have willingly and unknowingly entertained these voices and followed the distractions blindly.

All that matters is the choice you make right now, and each right now that follows. You are at the point of celebrating *that* you see, not judging *what* you see. So relax and enjoy the process. It can really be quite entertaining if you remember that you are becoming aware of the elaborate schemes by which you distract yourself from having the life that brings out the very best in you and fills you to the brim with joy. The voice of distraction is the voice of rationality run amok because it is not grounded in the clarity of heart's desire.

The basic point is that you have a Best Self. When you are quiet, you can hear the wisdom and truth it carries. Reconnecting with your Highest Self requires no "figuring out." The active mind is not required. The activity required is quieting the head to hear the heart. A preparation step for this part of the journey is to meet and greet the primary distraction(s) in your life and the various disguises it uses.

If your heart holds wisdom and truth, but you make your choices from your head without first consulting your heart as to whether a particular decision or choice nourishes or feeds the heart, you are on the path to closing your eyes and denying your power and splendor. For example, when you find a situation hysterically funny and suppress your humor because your head tells you that you need to appear serious and in control, you are denying the joy in your heart by not finding a way to express your laughter. If you do stop to ask what nourishes the heart, you will often find that the perspective you bring helps the entire situation in ways your head would not have recognized at the time. Likewise when you feel the inclination to stop for a few minutes, pour a cup of tea and listen to the rain on the roof, your heart is trying to signal what will serve you. Your head more often tells you to push yourself to be productive and get one more thing done. If you choose productivity, you close your eyes to your own joy and feed the pattern of making life more serious and difficult by not listening to your heart.

Don't look to society or social convention to help you. If you haven't noticed, the outside world is also asleep. Look to yourself, more specifically your heart, for clarity. A noisy head is the center of distraction from being present in your life. There are various reasons you might give your head such power. They are rooted in unexamined needs or desires that become distractions from life's path. Some of the most common are needs or desires:

- For approval or validation—looking externally to know that you are valued, that your choices are acceptable to others

- To prove yourself worthy—pleasing others, feeling worthy, good enough

- To belong and fit with a family, tribe, or other group—developing an identity through connection with others

- For control—seeking power over situations or others, being uncomfortable with the unpredictable and unknown

- To be right, to win, be successful—associating personal identity with knowing, having the "right" answers, measuring personal success by performance or achievements, being seen as smart

- To keep peace, preserve harmony—focusing primarily on others' comfort in relationships and situations, shutting down your own voice if you think that someone will be uncomfortable with something you might say or believe, avoiding conflict

- To be liked—ensuring that others know you have certain qualities, such as being responsible, dependable, nice, good, caring

Remember that unexamined conformity is a primary form of social control that distracts us from the joy and peace of our own paths. Who you are is not the same thing as what you do and therefore, not the same as the meanings that you assign to what you do. Watch carefully the voices in your head that tell you how to respond to situations, especially when your heart feels tight and your stomach churns at the thought of following that advice.

For example, if you want to see yourself as caring and believe that caring is a quality of your Highest Self, how you translate being caring into behavior must be weighed consciously by your own, and not society's truth meter.

  • Do you see yourself as caring because others have validated you for caring behaviors?

  • Might such a label cause you to engage in "taking care of" situations and other people when your body screams that you are too tired? Are you carrying others who are not choosing their own journey, playing instead on your sympathies?

  • Do you shut down your own truth when you think someone else might not feel cared for if you express your truth? Do you tell yourself that expressing and following your truth would be selfish and that service to others is noble, and listening to your own guidance is not?

The distraction pattern continues until you have to medicate yourself—in any of a variety of ways—to suppress feeling the frustration of not being seen and of making yourself smaller than you are so that others won't feel uncomfortable with the choice or expression that feels more true to you. Taking care of others at the cost of your voice and truth will eventually conflict with being your Highest Self and walking your path.

Caution: Ego identity can be hazardous to your path and full expression of your Highest Self.

The mask you wear to please others, gain acceptance or live into any other distraction is your ego identity. The danger comes from believing that you *are* the roles you fill and the qualities that you associate with successfully playing those roles. Being aware of the power you give to having certain qualities helps you to see how you distract yourself from your own gifts and joy.

Carefully examine how much of you and your behavior is actually driven by the external validation you receive for your choices. Do you feel joyful and fulfilled by your choices? Do you feel overwhelmed, exhausted, or maybe a little bit frustrated that you are the one doing the work? Just notice. No judgment. All you are looking at here is whether you are hearing your heart or listening to your head voices.

When you read the list of distractions, do you find a voice in your head judging or arguing with what is written? Are you inclined to rationalize why the statement might not apply to you? Do you find yourself saying, " Of course selfishness is the opposite of service?" Or perhaps, "What's so wrong with needing to be in control—that works for me and my life!"

Are you still denying that you distract yourself from being totally present to every moment in your life—fully engaged in the experience of the moment without analyzing, interpreting, questioning why or otherwise diverting your attention to the addictive power of your mind? Take an honest look at your schedule. Busyness is an earmark of a distracted life. How about the frequency with which you walk into your home and immediately turn on the television, radio, or music? When is the last time you turned off the iPod and listened to what was happening within your body as well as all around you? The heart's wisdom appears in silence; it does not compete with fillers or noise.

If you are tethered to technology, you are disconnected from your Highest Self. Still willing to open your eyes and tell yourself the truth? It means challenging some very deep patterns. These patterns don't currently serve your having the life big enough to support the Highest you and your potential. And, by the way, if you find yourself splitting hairs and qualifying the verbs I am using here—like claiming you are not "tethered," but are only "connected" to technology—that's a distraction of the mind, too.

When you are aware that something feels amiss, that you don't feel at the top of your game, you can begin the process of unraveling these unconscious distractions and their power over you. You can move towards reconnecting with your playful and lighthearted Highest Self. The vague sense that there must be more and something doesn't feel right is your heart voice getting through—however faintly—to wake you up. The next time you are feeling as though you just need to get through a task, stop and ask yourself whether you are spending large amounts of your days getting through tasks. If so, why? What messages do you listen to in your head to make yourself shut down your awareness that you are not having fun and that you want to be having fun? Place some funny picture or reminder on your mirror, desk, computer or other place where you look often to remind you to laugh. The reminder can serve as an honesty broker until you can make the changes in your life that support laughter and inspiration every day.

Let the critic voice go. Relax and get a kick out of how powerful your distractions are. They keep you living in such a state of doubt and fear that they have convinced you they are the only things you can trust. Know that you can let go of the string that holds them close at any time. When you are deeply connected to your truth and can hear the Inner Voice above the cacophony of voices in your head, it is much easier to release these distractions.

The theatre in your head has been playing the distractions non-stop, 24/7 three hundred sixty five days a year. And all along you thought the show was free! It has been costing you dearly and it is now time to open your eyes and make the choices that bring out the best in you—in your own time and in your own way. Realize that the theatre in your head is a torture chamber of "shoulds" with special roles for being productive, responsible, and nice. How much fun is that? Are you sure that you would rather be watching these continuous shows that constrain you in roles rather than listening to your wise and playful heart?

If you pause to ask whether the messages in your head fill you up, make your heart feel light, and give you energy, you can begin to recognize the difference between your truth and what outsiders have been telling you. You can begin to recognize which voices you listen to in your head that unconsciously judge success in life in terms of:

- Accomplishments

- Productivity

- Titles

- How many people's problems you solve

- How many voice or e-mails you get that tell you how important you are

Are you ready to consider *a whole new set of measures for success that are informed by your heart?* Consider the following heart measures:

- What brings you joy?

- When do you feel at peace, totally content to just *be*?

- How often do you respond to people or situations with appreciation and gratitude for what they bring, especially when it disrupts your plan for the situation?

- When you feel absolute abandon and lightness in life, what happens inside your chest or stomach?

- When you are filled with love, what moves you?

- When you are surrounded by Beauty, how do you respond?

- When you experience your own spaciousness, boldness, expansiveness, who do you become?

- What expression of your wisdom and truth sets you free and fills you with a sense of contribution and meaning?

Sit with these questions for a while. Come back to them. Roll them around until they feel comfortable and familiar. Don't push for answers. Let them come to you—maybe in the shower, or when you are not thinking specifically about them. Just sit with them. Take your time. When you want to know the answers, you are ready to begin In-Dwelling. That's the next step in moving away from the unconscious life of distractions to walk your path with ease. Clarity at the Center is the antidote to fear and doubt. Ready to go there?

In-Dwelling

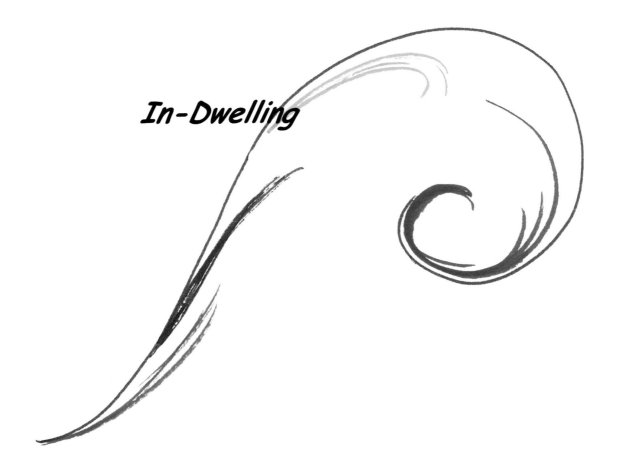

If you want to step into your own light and bask in the lightness and playfulness of who you truly are at your core, then it is time to clean house. The process of reconnecting with your Highest Self involves confronting each of the uninvited guest voices living in your head and deciding which ones are no longer welcome because in one way or another they are distracting you from seeing, touching, and feeling the beauty within. They are distracting you from your Inner Wisdom and truth. The process of shedding ideas, beliefs, attitudes, behaviors, and relationships that distract you from your Highest Self and unique path requires you to create stillness and quiet in your life so that you can hear your own truth above the voices in your head. This process is called in-dwelling.

To get started, think of the gentlest and kindest thing you could do for yourself and do it. Prepare to be nurtured and nourished. It has taken you many years, maybe even many decades to accumulate the distractions you have and it will take time, patience, and nurturance directed inward to release them. We are far better at accumulating, as a society, than at cleaning out and letting go. And believe me, once you get started, you won't want to stop. It can be exhilarating and unimaginably freeing to let go of what no longer serves you. As one client recently told me, "I could have never imagined that this one small step I avoided for so long could be such an enormous step in my feeling so light again!"

What may help you keep the big picture in focus is to create a metaphor for what in-dwelling is and does for you. You might think of in-dwelling as a process of building an addition onto your current house and sitting in it for a while until you sense what kind of space you want it to be and how you want it to look and feel. You are literally living into a part of you—the Center—that has been buried underneath the weight of daily distractions. As you travel on the Soul Grid, from the outer world of human rules, standards, and judgments back Home to reconnect with your Highest Self, you are engaging in a kind of conscious reflection about who you are today and what you hold onto that makes you who you are today.

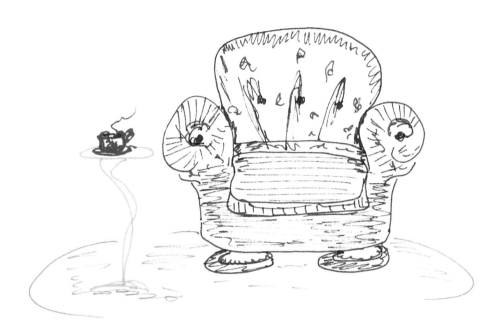

Another very powerful metaphor for not only the in-dwelling portion of your journey, but also the conscious living portion is the idea of creating and nurturing a splendid garden. You are designing the garden that is you, that expresses your gifts and qualities in ways that broadcast the beauty and brilliance within. When you pay attention to the vague sense of emptiness or dis-ease in your life, what you are really doing is focusing your intensity inward and listening to your own wisdom about what fills you with joy, peace, and passion and what drains you of the same. The work of the in-dwelling portion of growing this magnificent garden is readying the soil to both receive your gifts and also grow them into your highest potential, the fullest expression of your Highest Self. The soil must be ready for you to receive your heart's wisdom and know its truth and potential.

Preparing the Soil

• Survey the soil and location; see what exists today.

What this means is to look carefully at where you observe hardened and cracked soil because it has not been watered, or perhaps because it has "toughened up" to deal with situations and people who don't appreciate its magnificence. Perhaps your garden is trying to grow beautifully delicate flowers in an environment that will never sustain their growth. Maybe the garden consists of gorgeous tropical, bold, and colorful vegetation but the climate only supports ground cover and hearty plants. Whatever the case, it is time to notice what the condition of the soil is for growing all that is inside you that is ready to burst forth. In essence, you are surveying your receptivity for growth. Once you have taken note of the soil, you will need to recognize what kind of growth it is supporting. Are you fertile soil for love and support or do you protect yourself from (harden against) certain emotions, expressions of truth, or relationships? Is your soil filled with nutrients that support boldness and beauty or drained by relationships that are not returning the nutrients they take from the soil?

• Pay attention to what is growing and what is not. Weeds or flowers?

Is your life—garden—crowded by overgrowth of too many plants? Even if they are beautiful, there may be insufficient soil to nurture all of them. They end up competing against each other for nurturance. Or perhaps, the flowers that are true expressions of you are hemmed in and constrained by dense networks of roots and weeds that have crept into your garden and slowly overtaken the soil you need to express your Self. Why are weeds growing so easily in your garden?

• Devote the resources needed to prepare the soil for growth: remember that the root system is not visible on the surface and takes time to establish itself.

As you examine what is and is not growing and begin to clear away dense overgrowth, shed whatever you are growing that is not really you but which you have grown to please someone else. Recognize that the soil needs time to recover before you put anything else in it. It needs to be barren and empty for you to see the potential of the whole garden. You need to be able to step away, detach, and survey from a distance what wants growth and where and how that growth is best integrated in the plan for your garden. You need to remember that there is a natural rhythm in all of nature. There are seasons for clearing and seasons for growing.

We, humans, have a terrible habit of judging the absence of visible change as "nothing happening." When the soil is softening to receive the seeds, when the nutrients are being absorbed, when seeds are planted, it takes time before anything is really noticeable on the surface. A lot is going on—but we don't see it. Remember to foster the space for the root system to establish itself in the garden that is you. The in-dwelling process is a gradual and patient process that moves organically. Many things are going on long before you will be able to understand all that is growing within you. Patience and compassion for Self make the journey of discovery much more enjoyable.

As you think about creating the garden that is you, keep in mind that you are not planting a garden from scratch. The garden that represents your life as it is today has been growing for a long time, often without much attention to what is and what is not being watered and fed. Lots of weeding and pruning will be needed before any planting or transplanting is considered! That is the work of a very different process. For now the focus is only on preparing the soil for growth. In-dwelling requires great focus on the soil preparation phase of gardening and, therefore, conscious attention devoted to what wants growth and to creating the conditions to support that growth. It is a time for listening, a time for silence.

There is a time during which the soil is ready to receive seeds and a time when the ground is too hard. As you prepare the soil, you are also beginning to understand the timing and conditions for growth. You learn that just because you think it should be time for what you want to grow does not mean that the soil is ready. You may have to back up and watch for longer than you had thought. Enjoy it—and get out of your own way. If you have a high need to control things, practice controlling something else. You need your energy focused on noticing what is happening, because it is an absolute illusion to even think you are directing anything in this process.

When the soil is prepared to receive the seeds, you are reconnecting with the essence of the soil, your Center, and receptive to guidance about what to plant where. In effect, you have softened the ground to be open to your heart's Wisdom and intuitive guidance, the seeds of what you want to grow in your life. At the point where you have prepared the soil to receive intuitive guidance, doing the actual work of planting the seeds and tending the garden consciously leads you to reconnect with the beauty within you. As you prepare the soil in which to flourish, your focus inward helps you to carefully observe and listen to what wants growth, what grows naturally, and where you try to force growth that your garden does not support. At this point, you are on the path to understanding how your unique garden grows naturally and with ease.

What gardeners know that can help all of us flourish is that gardens don't just take care of themselves. If you don't remove leaves in the fall, they may flatten and snuff out whatever is growing underneath them. Clearing away the old is absolutely critical to make way for the new. You have to be discerning in weeding or you'll throw out new growth and flowers that haven't sprouted yet because you do not recognize the form they are taking. This one I learned as a child when my father asked me to weed the pansy bed, and I pulled up six yews he was growing from seed because they weren't pansies! It takes lots of time to weed the garden and prepare the soil to support new growth. The garden—the metaphor for our lives—moves on its own schedule! Give it space. You would give the space to your children or close friends as they move through life's transitions. Turn that same understanding inward and give it to your Self. After much time learning to do the same for myself—and a little gardening in the backyard, I wrote the following in my journal:

> *I actually enjoyed cleaning out the leaves, removing overgrowth, giving (the garden) a clean line... Cut away lots of overgrowth. Weeded out what I could but was disappointed not to be able to get to the roots of some and amazed at the density and networks of other weeds (not unlike the challenging of cherished beliefs and ways of operating that are pervasive, maybe even insidious—and definitely limiting growth in the spiritual garden).*

My Experience

> *Too much occupies my head. It's time to get quiet—and though earthly signals would say otherwise, it's time to go inward.*

Perhaps this is a good place to share with you how I got started on this whole process of in-dwelling. It goes back several years to a conversation with a teacher in my life who told me I needed to focus my intensity inward. I had absolutely no idea what she was talking about. But I did trust her guidance, because in the past she had seen patterns in my life that I needed to address to move into my own potential. I continuously seek that potential and know that I am generally comfortable trying new things that I don't fully understand. I guess it's a sense of discovery that beckons! I tend to listen to people whose wisdom I recognize as true for me and then try things I otherwise might not have considered on my own.

The conversation happened at a time in my life when I was vaguely aware that I was working very hard and not feeling particularly inspired. The business was going okay, but something felt vaguely unsatisfying or empty. If I was stuck, I was unaware of it—but that doesn't mean I wasn't stuck. It does mean that I was so desperately addicted to the speed and agility of my mind to address client issues to their satisfaction, that I had lost touch with what truly inspired me.

I was directed to spend three days in succession every month in silence. I could have music that was not distracting (no lyrics), but no other media. I could read about other people's journeys, but not about models, ideas, or theories. The notion of three days without clear outcomes or client meetings was completely foreign to me. My calendar was always booked months in advance. Yet I was told that three consecutive days were the minimum I would need to invest to do the work that was mine to do. I had no idea what that meant. I couldn't fathom how my being quiet and listening to myself could possibly yield anything of value, particularly since I had always found anything outside of myself to be infinitely more fascinating than anything inside me.

My initial questions were about how to be productive during those three days. What would I do? What should be happening? The purpose of the three days was to create quiet and focus inward. I could not know in advance what would happen because the inward journey would have been compromised. This exercise was about getting me to slow my life down and pay attention to what my inner life would reveal. This last statement had no meaning for me at the time. I was to commit the days, allow no outward distractions and notice what drew my attention. I was to quiet my head. A totally foreign concept at the time—and not one I was even sure I valued!

The voices of self-doubt in my head, unconsciously internalized over a period of years, were loud. They were reinforced by people in my life who thought that what I was doing—and why I would not be available to talk with them for three days—was a bit absurd. Nevertheless, I trusted the advisor who told me to get quiet and see what happened. As a small business owner who only generated revenue when I did something for clients, I needed to address with my business partner that I would be taking three business days each month to be silent. Luckily, she was supportive, although skeptical of my willingness to blindly follow a directive to set aside three days for an unspecified time to achieve something that was not—and could not be—explicitly clear. I felt intrigued by the challenge and was not at all hesitant about setting aside the time, even though I could not articulate why. I know, in retrospect, that my intuition was prompting me to try the process.

I blocked three days on my calendar every month through the end of the year. I told my business partner and parents that I would be unavailable to them three days every month. To others I gave no explanation. I began the process of being quiet and keeping a journal about what I was thinking and feeling. I did things like wander around the house, garden, go for walks, do art work, and read about the journeys of wise teachers. The process of in-dwelling was completely foreign to me. Nothing felt familiar. I could not make meaning about what I was doing or even what the goal might be. I had some vague sense that something very important would reveal itself, and that I could not know it as I went into the process. I later understood that that vague sense was the very Wisdom I usually allowed my head to override.

I knew that what I was undertaking was important and that it was going to feel different and unfamiliar. I also knew that I was not to focus on "productivity" at any level, if the process were to be successful. It was about creating fertile soil to grow. This was the beginning of the preparation of the soil. Instead of a hard-driving mental focus on helping clients address challenges, I was to soften the soil so that I could connect better with my heart and intuition. I had no idea what to do during my three days except to surround myself with what nourished me—and even that took time to recognize. I set about creating three days of silence every month for nearly three years. And though I typically offered no explanation, clients and colleagues learned to deal with the fact that my usual policy of responding to requests within twenty-four hours would sometimes break down.

The results were astounding in their depth and simplicity. I rediscovered who I am at my Center and developed the clarity and courage to make changes in my life that support my Highest Self. Today I lead much more from my heart. I am acutely aware of where I invest my energy and whether what comes back to me is worth the investment. I am aware of when I am inspired by my work, my interactions, and my relationships—and of what I need to change when I am not. I more often recognize my intuition as it is speaking to me.

My journey, and the three days of in-dwelling each month are unique to me. Part of what I was to do through in-dwelling was to reconnect with my Highest Self. The other part was to listen to the Wisdom about how to help others do the same thing. When I created the space and intention to hear my Inner Voice, I came to understand our collective and individual paths more clearly. I came to understand the Universal Soul Grid and patterns that give meaning to the apparent chaos in our lives. I had to develop a powerful relationship with space and silence to recognize them as comforts and sources of security in my life and to discover the Wisdom within.

However much time you need to set aside, know that there is nothing magical about allocating exactly and only three days each month. That was what I needed to do because I was so incredibly unconscious and the structure of my life would not have allowed me to do the inner work I needed to do without a significant "time out" on a regular basis. Part of my work involved my experiencing in-dwelling so consciously that I could understand how to teach it to others.

Your path is likely to be very different. Why you need to go inward and what wisdom awaits you inside is for you to discover. All I can offer you at this point is that your commitment to stepping into your brilliance and light will guide you to listen to how much time, with what frequency, spent in what location will create the space for you to genuinely crave more time to go inward. As I intersperse tips from my own journey, I also offer direct reflections and insights that I recorded in journals over the three-year period. They are captured in italics, as they came to me in my own process. The language may sound odd or "out there" at times, but I have tried to remain true to sharing with you how I came to recognize my Inner Voice. Enough about me. Let's shift the focus to the in-dwelling process itself.

The *in-dwelling process* follows three critical steps:

- Create the space to go inward
- Shine the light on unconscious patterns and behaviors
- Discern Inner Wisdom from noise

Let's begin with the first step.

Create the Space to Go Inward

What does this mean? The intensity you currently focus on the needs of everyone else around you, arranging your life around demands at work and every other priority that leaves no room for you to just be quiet with nothing to do for anyone else, needs to be turned inward. Like most everything else in life, this is not a matter of shutting your current life off and trading it in for a new one immediately—although some of you might like this option!

It is about making the commitment to discover your inner space, to live in your heart with no distractions for some period of time that you choose on a regular basis. There is a lot of room for flexibility here for what can work and how this can look within the context of your current life.

Coach's tip: What's required to be on the journey, in the dance, is commitment.

This means that anyone who chooses to live into his or her highest potential can engage the journey. It is very doable. Watch the voices in your head that tell you this is impractical, some kind of New Age hoo hah, or that it is a waste of time. The job of the ego—your identity with what you do—is to preserve the status quo, to preserve favored child status for the head, which has been ruling your kingdom for a long time. The heart is ready to share its wisdom. Are you ready to do what it takes to create some space in your life to hear it?

Brian Andreas captures what happens when we refuse to listen to our Inner Wisdom in his poem, "Hearing Voices."[1]

> I used to hear
> voices a lot,
> but then I read
> up on it &
> found out
> they don't exist
> > so now I don't
> > listen to a word
> > they say

We have given our power to external sources without checking out their credentials and loyalties to make decisions that truly serve us. How logical is that? No wonder our gardens are overgrown with weeds!

So—How do you create the space in your life to go inward?

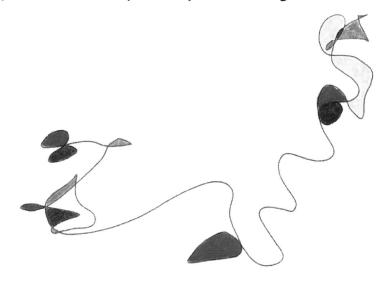

Here are four tips that will help:

a. Give yourself permission to create quiet space and do it
b. Detach from a focus on "doing"
c. Experience and pay attention to feelings and reactions
d. Get comfortable with and build nurturing structures

Let's spend some time with each of these points to see how they actually play out in developing your process for in-dwelling.

Give yourself permission to create quiet space and do it

Consciously giving yourself permission to create the time and space to be still, quiet, is critical. Recognize early on that you can't know what the outcome of in-dwelling will be. That means you don't have the perfect answer for others who want your time and attention. Make it easy on yourself. Allocate time in your schedule in a way that you don't have to deal with others' expectations of your availability to them. For example, if you are a parent of young children, consider giving yourself thirty minutes when the kids are napping to not answer the telephone—take it off the hook or turn it off. Sit in your favorite spot and be comfortable. If you are at some kind of office job every day, enter a "telephone conference" on your calendar on a regular basis every week or create the name for a meeting that you will actually keep. You may find that the easiest time to start this process is at the beginning of the workday, lunch, or end of the day.

If there is any way possible, leave the physical place where you do your work in order to clear your head. Consider walking outside the building, or going to another floor. The whole idea is for you to give yourself permission to create space to be quiet. Many people find it helpful to get up early or to let the family know that for some period of time in the evening, they are not available. Even if it is for the length of time of a shower or bath, find time and physical space for just you.

For this process to work, you actually have to see your relationship with Self as one of the critical relationships in your life. This may feel odd, since it has likely been a neglected one for a very long time. In-dwelling involves an initial step of creating a space—physical and emotional—separate from your regular routine. You will know what you need to truly nurture your Self as you engage in the process. It's like buying a wonderful new abode and decorating it just for you, having everything present in color, style, music, smells, sights, and sounds that nurture your Soul—everything that delights you. This is not a time of denying your Self what nurtures you. The space you create within your life for in-dwelling is to be a place of celebration that invites and envelops you. It is a sanctuary just for you.

I am appreciating going inward. I am loving the cozy space where in-dwelling abides. It is warm, comforting, asks only that I show up and enjoy its gifts.

Such a place provides a haven where you remove the familiar markings, touchstones, and structures with which you construct your daily life. No telephone, blackberry, e-mail, or television. No outside voices of any kind that would distract you from going inward and learning to wait for what emerges. For some people stillness is a foreign experience and one they often avoid at all cost. When you are ready, stillness is not scary; it is comforting and nurturing.

My journey absolutely requires me to slow down to focus the intensity on a narrower band when I go inward...shift from extending energy broadly—expansively to focusing it deeply and thoroughly.

You may find, as I did, that a kind of walking meditation helps. Walking meditation is where you quiet your mind from thinking about all you need to do in the future or preoccupying your mind with concerns from the past. You focus instead on your breathing, or pay attention to what you see, hear, smell, and feel as you walk. Physical activity, such as yoga, tai chi, or walking on a beach, allows you to become more present and to really notice your physical body's response to each moment. In-dwelling is about removing the outside distractions so that you can be fully aware of what is happening, and what you are experiencing in every moment, as it happens. It's not about analyzing or making meaning of what you experience. It is about being very quiet and fully engrossed in whatever you are experiencing. All mental activity is directed towards noticing, including noticing what you are noticing!

Everybody has an excuse for why he or she cannot do it now. What is yours? Bad time at work? It's not a good time for your spouse, partner, or lover? Can't do it while the kids are still at home? You're the only one who can do something that needs to be done?

Listen to your litany of excuses for how busy you are. Today's excuse is one thing. Tomorrow's excuse will be another. There is never a perfect time. You must make time, as you would for anything else in your life that you decide is important to you. If you really want to create time to find out who is at your Center, what a life of Grace would offer you, make the decision to go inward—and stick with it. If not, don't, because half way in doesn't work.

Once you have made the commitment to create quiet, you will have plenty of company with the voices in your head that find this decision foreign and want to distract you from your quiet. You will become acutely aware of your head yammering at you that "this is stupid," or "this isn't productive." By making quiet space a regular part of your life—like brushing your teeth or combing your hair—you will begin to notice how much and about what subjects you engage to daydream, fantasize, plan, or relive the past.

In-dwelling will make you acutely aware of all the escape strategies you typically use to avoid feeling what is real in any given moment. This new focus inward also makes it easier for you to consciously know what is real in the moment as opposed to a distraction of the mind.

If someone close to you calls to ask you to cover for him so that he can honor another commitment and the time he is asking for is your time to be quiet, will you remember the promise you made to yourself? Or will you tell yourself that you can take care of yourself any time and he needs you now? This kind of thinking is a trap and it is how you got to where you are today. You know that what he is asking you to do is not how you need or want to be spending your time. The more you hold the intention to create quiet to discover your Highest Self, the more you will be able to recognize the voices in your head for what they are—distractions from what is real in the moment. You might discover that you are only responding out of guilt or fear of disappointing someone—both distractions from Highest Self. A more honest and real response might be to let the caller know that you have other plans and will not be available to help him this time. No more explanation is needed. Then notice how your body responds when you listen from within. Do you relax or tighten up? Does your stomach churn or do you experience some relief? Don't analyze anything. Just pay attention.

Remember that it's about preparing the soil for the garden to flourish. We are a culture that wants the garden to sprout immediately. It won't work that way. There's a natural rhythm in nature, and it's not going to change because you have decided you don't have time to wait. It takes nine months to make a baby, whether you want it to or not. Prepare the soil. Prepare to be more intrigued by discovering how things actually evolve than by trying to control them. Nurture patience because you care enough to receive the wisdom that comes from staying on the inward path. You are building your capacity to hear your Inner Wisdom, the heart's truth about what wants to grow within you and about what aspects of your Self you have shut down.

When we recognize that what is called for is a journey inward, a change in the status quo, that is precisely the point in our lives where we sabotage our own journey, where we avoid turning inward because we are terrified. We intuitively know that change is afoot and instead of going gracefully and allowing the path to reveal itself, we fight it. We work harder at making a less than satisfying job, relationship, or idea "work" rather than listening as every cell in our bodies tells us that it is no longer working for us. It no longer—if it ever did—brings satisfaction and joy.

There are two strong clues that warn us that we are not ready or don't want to venture inward:

- Telling our Selves that we don't have time
- Telling our Selves that we don't have the money

We can find every reason to justify why we cannot take the time away from work or family. Time and money are distractions. They are ways we keep ourselves from heeding the heart's Wisdom and re-engaging that Wisdom to direct our lives. Be honest with yourself. If there is something you passionately want in life—more than anything—you figure out how to make the time. If you don't have the money, you will figure out how to barter or otherwise creatively finance what you want. The real question is whether you want to discover the brilliant gem inside—Highest Self—and live your life easily creating the life you want. It is within the reach of the humblest. And it requires only your commitment.

So if you are ready, and you are willing to be invited into the inner chambers where you keep the secrets even you do not remember hiding about your passions and what you love, then set aside time that is yours alone. That is all that is asked to begin the journey. Demonstrate that you are committed to reconnecting with your passions and more expansive Self by scheduling time. Time to just **be**. Time to be very present to whatever comes your way. Time to be open and gentle with yourself. Time to be quiet. Preparing the soil is the first step on the path to seeing what fosters your gifts and where you shut your Self down. You already know it is time to change, but you may not consciously know what that entails, where and how you need to move, or what will cause you to feel more complete and more joyful.

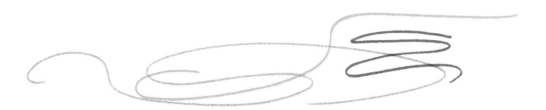

Coach's Tip: Put time on your calendar in a way that you do not feel inclined to explain to others why or that you are not available to them. Do not invite questions. Declare this time "already booked."

At the point where you can trust a vague sense of knowing that something needs to change, you are ready to become more reflective, to notice your response to what happens each day, to each person you encounter. It is a time of paying attention to what your body tells you. When a situation presents itself, does your chest get tight, does your stomach churn, do your palms sweat? Pay attention. The Wisdom within is trying to get your attention, trying to help you discern the direction or choice that might best serve you at this point. At the same time, your ego—your head voice—is invested in maintaining the status quo. It will work twice as hard and many times faster to convince you that things are fine and you don't have time for "this stuff." Focus on the body messages instead, stepping back enough to understand that your heart messages about what is true for you, which decisions support your Highest Self and which distract you are registering in your body. Pay attention to what decisions feel freeing and which ones feel heavy or constraining.

The outside voices and relationships that shape and reward you for being who you are today and making the choices you do, are invested in your not changing. Truth comes from within. When you make the commitment to listen to what is true for you, you can finally act on that truth, rather than distracting your Self to please others. Deep in the center of your truth lies the clarity of your heart's passion and the best in you. The first step in discovering and rediscovering your passion and Highest Self is creating the time and space in your life to go inward. Do it regularly to reconnect with your Highest Self.

Be quiet and listen. The answers are in the silence.

Now that the time is on the calendar, you are ready for the second critical step in creating the space to go inward:

Detach from a focus on "doing"

There's a fun one! What does this mean? This concept is foreign in Western culture. We might be more aptly named "human doings" if you really look at our behavior and priorities today. When you consider carpools, hours at work, time at the gym or working out, meetings, and the myriad of other things occupying every moment of our time, there is no such thing as "down time" or silence, unless we consciously create it.

Early on in your in-dwelling process, it is very important to let go of any need to feel that the time you spend in silence be "productive." The drive for productivity is a head distraction that we have bought into as a society. Closer examination will reveal that it overrides the wisdom of the heart. The heart would guide us to do less and to do so in ways that create joy and a more peaceful way of living. Instead of being exhausted and short with people because we are trying to get one more thing done before the day ends, we might actually hear the child's laughter and join in. We might respond spontaneously to a desire to watch the stars rather than some mindless show on television that is keeping us company while we finish reading the paper or e-mail messages.

Once you let go of the expectation that you need to be productive in the space you have created, you are ready to let go of the need to be "doing" anything! We tend to determine our lives' success and meaning today by some measure of how busy we are. Doing nothing but being present and paying attention to how you feel and what you are experiencing gives new purpose to using the space you have created. You become aware of how much of your identity, your ego, is tied to who needs you, and how many phone calls or e-mails await your reply. Be careful—it's a trap! When who you are equals what you do, the voice of your Highest Self is absent. When you find yourself tethered to work, another person, or some form of technology every waking moment, it is time to step back and notice how the addiction to doing and feeling connected is sucking the life out of you.

If only for a brief period of time in your busy schedule, you have to abandon your need to define your worth or value by what you are doing or what you have accomplished in your quiet time. For a while you will not see any "results" because it takes time to prepare the soil and what is happening is happening so deeply within you that you do not yet have the capacity to see it. If you are not ready to let go, you are not ready to go inward. You can't find Wisdom if it can't find you. And it cannot find you if you're buried in a schedule that allows no space for quiet and reflection. It can find you when you are doing nothing but being present. No more is asked. No more is needed to go inward.

The detachment from expectation, willingness to experience, and full engagement in silence clears out the noise and distraction. It creates a space that is both enormously full and empty.

So what does it look like when you are not focused on being productive, when you are not focused on doing anything, and when you have created a space to be quiet? What is happening?

What you are doing at this point is really creating a physically comfortable place in which to be quiet. Where can you be that you will not be disturbed and where you feel nurtured, cared for, and treated to time with yourself? Hint: It does not have any other people in it! So—it is not going to a class where you learn something, even if it's about something you love. This is not a time for putting anything into your head. This is a time to get stuff out!

Is the space outside in nature or inside? Whatever supports stillness is the answer. You might be inside listening to the rain on the roof or watching the waves at the beach. Do you need to stay in one space the whole time? No! But you do need to be quiet. Walking is a great activity. Paying attention to everything around you when you walk and noticing when thoughts pop into your head is helpful. Allowing yourself to wonder about who you become when you feel light and unburdened or what makes you most joyful makes it easier to stay open to what you notice. The answers will not be "head words" like "organized, plays well with others, and delivers results on time."

Your Highest Self has no connection to obligations, shoulds, what is noble, burdens or heaviness. It is light and lighthearted. What that feels and looks like for you is unique to you. But fundamentally, Highest Self is playful—and loves it! What do you *love* about you? Are you vibrant? Bold? Wacky? Spontaneous? Do you have a great sense of humor? Do you love to dance? Sing? Twirl with complete abandon? Here is an exercise many people have found helpful to get started in reconnecting with Highest Self.

CREATING SPACE TO JUST *BE* EXERCISE

Find a comfortable chair in a place where you will not be disturbed. Have paper and pen nearby.

- Think back to the specific things that brought a smile to your face, delight to your heart, and a giggle or laugh out loud as a child.

- Make a list of your favorite things.

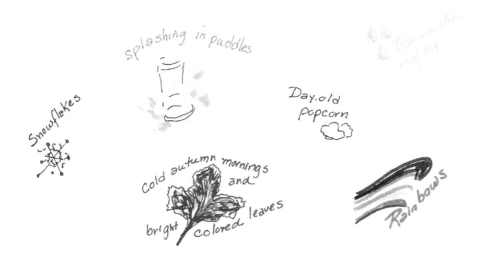

- Whatever is on that list, add to it what brings that same smile, laughter and delight today.

- Sit with this list. Really allow it to fill you up. Then quietly notice how you feel when you are filled with these things.

- Do you find an overwhelming sense of fulfillment, peace, joy?

- What do you feel like doing?

- What qualities does being filled with these things bring out in you? Do you feel relaxed or energized? Quiet or loud?

- Are you inclined to do something or be silent?

- What pops into your head when you fill yourself with what you love?

Keep written notes about what you notice. You can repeat this exercise any time by simply recalling your favorite things and allowing them to fill you up.

Here is another exercise that can help you be aware of where you are focusing your energy and what you experience in return.

ENERGY TRACKING EXERCISE

Wherever you find yourself, pay attention to people, places, things, relationships, and ideas at the same time as you notice body signals. Notice:

What gives you energy?

What drains your energy?

If you pay attention to only these two questions, you will be doing the work of creating the space to be present in your life. You will also be building your capacity to discern what supports your Highest Self and what constrains or shuts it down. Take the time to really notice...over...and over again, until you are constantly noticing which environments, relationships, ideas, and conversations in your life are filling you up and which ones are wearing the Best in you down.

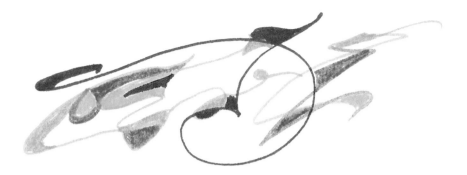

In the early stages of creating the space and clearing the noise, you may find that you are looking for things to do. Notice when you do this, what you choose to do or not do, and how you experience the time and engagement with whatever you attempt to do. Initially, some activities may be fun or relaxing. You may enjoy some form of physical movement—such as walking or hiking—or meditating, or creating some form of artistic expression, or watching ducks on a pond. Whatever you choose to do, notice how you make the choice to do it and how you experience the activity. Remember that the activity needs to support you in being silent and solitary, while still feeling nurtured.

Once you practice in-dwelling for a period of time that establishes some regularity in your life, you may notice that you feel less need to be doing anything at all. Time will slow down and you will slow down with it, experiencing less and less inclination to schedule or plan anything. Even if the activities you are planning are what you love, you will begin to notice that you don't want to plan anything and in the moment, do not want to do what you had planned. Listen to your heart and follow its direction. Let whatever you feel in the moment shape what you choose to do.

The vast majority of things you find yourself doing because you thought you would love to have the time to do them may begin to feel like obligations. It sounds funny at the beginning, but this shift in perception does happen. You may find that if you are totally present, with no plans to do anything, something will come to you that is exactly what fills you at the time.

If you accept the mental distraction of planning to do activities because you said you would, you will slow your journey inward. Instead begin to notice how much the thought forms that pop into your head can interfere with your ability to connect with your heart. For every present moment where you remove yourself from what you are experiencing in the moment to entertain an idea in your head—about what you had planned to do, or how long you had planned to spend doing something, or what order you had planned your activities—you are detaching from hearing your heart's wisdom about what you deeply want and feel in that moment. You must be entirely present to both fully touch each moment and allow the beauty of each moment to touch you.

> *It doesn't really matter what I do but my level of consciousness, presence and awareness does. How intentional I am to be quiet, empty, open to explore inner space is critical. These days I find thoughts of work during (in-dwelling) less intrusive, less present.*

For those wanting to find this place of inner wisdom, the in-dwelling time and space in your life begin to feel like precious gifts. As with the beginning of any new activity, there is an initial phase where practicing the new way feels very unnatural and you will be tempted to give up on it. Your unconscious patterns of distraction, such as mind wanderings and fantasies about how you want things to play out, draw your attention away from focusing inward. They fill your silence with noise. You may find it helpful to reframe the journey inward in some way that reminds you that you are choosing in-dwelling. Take care to remind yourself of the desire to be in touch with your heart's wisdom, in a way that supports patience and curiosity, and allows you to recognize and dismiss distractions. One way to do this is to consciously say aloud, "Fantastic! I've got thirty minutes just for me to be and do whatever fills me." In effect, you are telling your mind to wait for thirty minutes before interrupting because you are busy in-dwelling. When your head is leading your life, your Best Self is missing. Consciously commit to listening to your heart so that it can lead. Commitment to rediscovering your passion, knowing what is really important to you, and hearing the Wisdom of your heart can reel you back from the jaws of distraction and prepare you to appreciate each moment. The following exercise may help.

PROMPTS TO GET MORE PRESENT EXERCISE

The prompts that follow are designed to help you focus your attention on your sensory experience—hearing, sight, touch, smell—in order to quiet your mind. You may choose to use each prompt independently or consider combining some. Whatever helps you to shift your focus to your experience of the moment over the thoughts in your mind is what works for you.

Notice what happens when you turn off all noise in your house or room.

- Try coming home and not turning on the radio, stereo, television, or any other form of technology.
- Alternatively, when you get in your car to go anywhere, try paying complete attention to what you see, hear, and experience without turning on the radio or CD in the car.
- Distance yourself from anticipating what you will find when you get wherever you are going and stay present with what you notice as you drive.
- What do you hear or see?
- Try listening so carefully that you can hear beyond the noise to silence. (This activity may take some practice!)

When you listen to the quiet, notice how your body responds.

- Is your chest tight or open?
- Is your jaw relaxed?
- How about your stomach?

When you go outside, notice what you experience and which senses command your attention.

- Do you feel the air when you go outside? Do you notice its temperature?
- What does the ground feel like under your feet? Stand still for a moment and notice what happens.

- What do you hear outside? Listen more.
- What do you smell?
- Try balancing on one foot. How does this activity shift your focus?   What do you notice?

Something you can do inside or outside is to stop, be quiet and pay attention to your own breathing.

- Is it shallow or deep—from the diaphragm?
- Try counting each breath and notice where and when you lose count.

You can use this prompt anytime to reduce stress in the moment.

Notice colors and shapes and don't be afraid to lose yourself in watching them and how they change.

- For example, notice patterns and shapes of clouds. How are they moving in the sky?
- Water and fire are just as fascinating to watch.
- Notice your breath while watching either one for even five minutes.
- Pay attention to how your body responds as you focus on the patterns and colors you see.

The point of the prompts is to begin to bring your Self back to the present moment to really experience—not to analyze, interpret, or judge—what is happening. It is a critical step in creating quiet space and in developing your capacity to detach your identity from "doing". You are building your capacity to watch your Self as you experience life.

Preparation of the soil to receive Wisdom takes time and practice. It is a time for compassion. This is not a time to deny yourself the simple pleasures that relax you—a cup of tea, a cozy chair, sunlight on your face. ***The notion that in-dwelling to develop a more conscious life path must be spartan or austere is simply false and unproductive.*** You are consciously preparing a space in which to discover riches. That means that the space must be desirable—or you won't want to go there emotionally or physically.   Remember that in-dwelling is a gift and not a punishment. It is a reward you give your Self once you realize that you want to contribute from your highest potential and feel the power of your own light.

If you are ambivalent about creating space or inclined to try in-dwelling so that you can check it off your list or join the "flavor-or the month" club, don't even bother. You will be inclined to do the exercises half way or not at all. It won't take long before you allow any outside demand to become more important than the investment in your own potential. I'll save you the trouble. For you, the process won't work, simply because you are not yet ready—you arc not focused or committed enough to its success to follow the process. No judgment. Be both honest and patient with yourself. Admit that you are not ready and come back to it when you are.

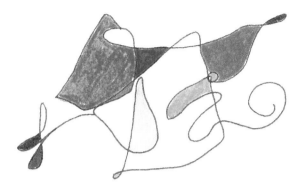

There are many ways you can tailor your own process to fit your life. There are also a few requirements. Creating space and detaching from doing are two of them. Building the capacity for even more silence is essential. You have to make your own soil preparation a worthy focus in your life in order to continue.

For those that give into doubt or run back to other people for approval and reasons to support why such an effort is not appropriate "at this time," you may find a pattern of slow, difficult, or painful transitions in your life. Some people seem to saunter through life and the changes it presents. Others go kicking and screaming, sometimes feeling like they walk down the street with a cloud over their heads. Which of these descriptions more closely resembles you?

Coach's Tip:
If you believe you must go through suffering and pain to move to enlightenment, then that will be the experience you create.

If you choose to walk in light and stay awake to whatever presents itself to you in your life, then that will be the experience you create.

Remember that you are the one putting all the interpretation and meaning into whatever you encounter in your life. You are creating the experience you have.

When you are at the point where you are defining success in human terms—things, money, titles—and are feeling stuck or vaguely unfulfilled, it is time to really pay attention to what brings you joy and what you find to be easy versus difficult in life. The signals of joy are the small lights in your life that represent your heart's voice. Look carefully for each of them. They are there. They may be small or infrequent, but they are there. It is time to reconnect with your inner truth about what fills you up rather than external definitions of success that trigger a sense of obligation or "should."

What is happening is that you have learned what it takes to be successful by societal or other external measures, but your Highest Self is not being nurtured. The vague sense of emptiness or general malaise is the signal that it is time to shift your focus inward in order to reclaim your true voice and gifts and to follow your unique path. On the Soul Grid, you are at the Away spiral being prompted to look inward, to engage that journey to hear your inner voice, your heart, over the voices in your head. It is time to engage the process of in-dwelling. It is a time of unraveling the path you have traveled outward, the path of expansion into new roles and focus on people and things outside your Self. It is a time to return Home—with your eyes wide open—to who you are at your Center.

As you unravel what you have unconsciously picked up along the way while acquiring your ego-identity, you consciously see what values your choices now reflect, what relationships take more from you than you get back, what you have incorporated and how disconnected you are from your passion and heart's true desires. The awakening that occurs when you consciously experience silence eventually overrides any sense of Self that comes from "doing". You are only just preparing the soil for this Highest Self to more fully express itself. Once you have created space and begun to focus on detaching your identity from what you do, the next part of really living into the space is to develop your capacity to be very present in all aspects of your life. What will help you to more fully experience the space you are creating now is to:

Experience and pay attention to feelings and reactions

Along the in-between from the known pattern is a stage of transition, which seems without shape or clear direction...without perspective it can feel chaotic or stuck.

Along the path inward, once you have committed to engaging the journey, you will begin to experience the unfamiliar. You begin to notice your body's signals of discomfort when you make choices that neglect your Highest Self in order to lead the life validated by those outside you. The process of becoming aware of your heart's tugs and truth can feel like wearing new shoes. When they are new, you notice they are a little stiff, where they crease, where they pinch, and where the fit is right. Until the shoes feel familiar and comfortable on your feet, you pay attention. You notice the fit. So, too, with the patterns and relationships which shape your life.

What is new gets your attention until you relax into its patterns and then they become familiar to you. You engage them automatically, without noticing or thinking. It is far easier to learn something new than to unlearn something unconscious, much easier to accumulate than to discard. So be kind to yourself. You are becoming aware of just how much you have been accumulating and carrying in your life so far. You are feeling the weight of all you have unconsciously chosen to carry without realizing that it has been your choice to carry it all along. The in-dwelling process is one of reflecting on what you are carrying and what does and does not fill you. You are developing the capacity to more easily shed whatever does not serve the Best in you by becoming more aware.

Getting rid of stubborn patterns of thinking is not for sissies! Being able to recognize and call attention to patterns that are automatic—where no actual thinking occurs—as when you drive through the traffic light and then ask yourself whether it was green when you went through—requires commitment and persistence. The work is invasive and thoughtful, time consuming, and demanding of your undivided attention. It is also an opportunity to engage your sense of adventure and discovery.

I remember a time when I was in my art studio, playing with clay. I was much more familiar with drawing and sketching. I had not worked with clay and was literally just playing with what it felt like to work in three dimensions. I thought about what I wanted to make with the clay I held in my hands. But something else happened.

I didn't think clay was my medium because I thought I didn't know how to make certain things...I guess that's not a problem when it sculpts itself! And the form seemed to come out of nowhere. I had no idea in my head to sculpt a bird.

A bird is what I formed. Not because I consciously knew how to make a bird, but because when I was very quiet and simply playing with the clay, I naturally created a bird. I noticed that when I told myself that clay was not my medium, sculpting wasn't fun. I didn't enjoy the process and I was extremely critical of the result. I had thought I wanted to make something else and when my creation did not take form, as I wanted it to, I decided I wasn't good at sculpting.

Once I became more conscious of how I was approaching the whole process of creating something with clay, I could see how the way I was thinking about my relationship with clay mirrored other patterns in my life. I became more consciously aware of ways by which I create my own stress. I learned how performance expectations, that I set, rob me of thoroughly engaging in a purely joyful discovery process. I began to comprehend the cost of being attached to expectations and results.

Coach's tip: Pay attention to points in your life where you get bent out of shape because the outcome you wanted didn't happen.

If you are unconscious about what kind of meaning you attach to situations and how you frame or label them, you are destined to create expectations that limit your ability to just enjoy what presents itself. For example, imagine having an identity that is tied to always doing the "responsible" thing. You might find that you are unable to enjoy group activities where there is potential risk that someone might get hurt—because you would feel responsible. Since you feel obliged to live up to your identity as the responsible one in the group, you plan for the ideal outcome and are constantly watching for what might go wrong. You are not present to enjoy the experience at all. You would like to be able to enjoy the activity but have created a situation where the group is counting on you to make sure everything is safely planned and no one gets hurt.

Your assumed ego identity in the group becomes a distraction from who you would like to be and what you would like to be doing with your energy and gifts. Over time your attachment to being responsible becomes so ingrained that you are unaware of how disconnected you are from your path and passion. You are only aware of being unfulfilled. Your assumptions about what nourishes your soul and how that happens are skewed, if not total delusions. You develop a pattern of convincing yourself that this is your role, others are counting on you, and you have no choice. You learn—unconsciously—to lie to yourself about how good your choices make you feel in order to keep choosing the ego identity of being responsible over feeling free. This is the price of becoming the ego identity you have built for your Self!

The antidote to such unconscious attention to living into the identity you have built for your Self is to step back and watch your Self in various situations. Conscious attention paid to your physical sensations and feelings in every present moment helps you to be more honest with your Self about what is actually happening. It also gives you an opportunity to create the space where your Inner Voice—via body signals or other means—is heard above the din of other voices in your head. With practice, it becomes easier to create that space, because you become consciously aware of your body's response, your emotional reactions, and any other kinds of responses to thoughts, situations, or people you encounter in the moment.

Developing a conscious awareness of how you are reacting at any given moment is an important step in cultivating the space to hear your own Inner Wisdom. Your body will signal you when you are on track, when something feels right, or when you are forcing something you don't really want or that doesn't support your truth. Pay attention to your body and to where you register reactions physically in your body. Is it in your stomach, or does your chest get tight? Does your heart get heavy? Does your throat clamp down and get dry? Do you tend towards headaches or back pain? Is your life full of "pains in the neck" or "pains in the ass?" Is there some part of your back that tenses up? How about weight on your shoulders or tightness in your jaw? Notice where, in your body, you first register signals related to what you are thinking or deciding at the time. Notice how a specific decision makes you feel.

Pay particular attention to whether your head wants to assign these sensations or physical reactions an emotional label such as, "I'm feeling sad." The head may also judge the sensation: "That doesn't mean anything. I'm overreacting." Remind yourself that the ego identity's job is to preserve the status quo, the old patterns. Your mind doesn't like recognizing that it is not in control of something new that you are choosing. The familiar unconscious patterns that you are releasing are head distractions from the Wisdom of the heart that lives—albeit neglected—deep within. Your Inner Voice speaks the heart's Wisdom, and it is buried under the weight of the voices in your head at any given time.

You may find the following exercise helpful in noticing where your head attempts to interfere with your body's messages. This exercise can be applied to any kind of physical activity. The illustration here uses yoga.

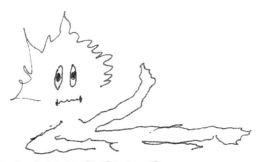

LISTENING TO YOUR BODY EXERCISE

Consider using a yoga CD or tape to practice paying attention to your body.

- Notice, as you learn poses, how your head wants to judge their relative difficulty.

- Notice where you impose your willpower to go beyond where you body is comfortable.

Then stop and gently give your body something it needs—back off. Get rid of the competitive performance-based or perfection need to do the pose as the instructor does it.

- Listen to and feel what your body wants to do. Pay attention.

- Stay with the pose and wait until something moves and you can shift into the position a bit more.

In that moment notice what happens when you work with the wisdom of your body, and don't attempt to override it with judgments from your head and further imposition of your will.

If you practice listening and feeling what your body is ready to do, you can develop the capacity to notice where you are forcing things in other parts of your life, rather than trusting what feels right in the moment. *It is the difference between knowing what you want and forcing it to happen and knowing what you want and watching for opportunities for it to happen easily and naturally.* This exercise can help attune you to the difference. The former takes a lot of effort and energy; the latter is effortless.

As you pay more attention to whatever you are experiencing, notice what stands out for you. Keep track of observations without judging them. When I was first beginning my own process of in-dwelling, I kept a journal of what I was noticing. Here are some examples of early observations:

I notice how literally I respond to something new.

I feel a need to conserve energy, though my head wants to "do" something.

Music is a huge part of my Soul connection. It takes me right out of my head and brings me present.

Notice that there is no judgment of worth in any of these statements. It is not that what you notice is necessarily good or bad, effective or ineffective in the situation you are experiencing. What is happening in this phase of creating the space to go inward is that you are beginning to actually see and recognize the thinking and behavioral patterns that you unconsciously engage on a regular basis. You may begin to notice choices that you hadn't previously recognized as choices. For example, you may be one who ignores body signals to slow down until you are stopped by illness or complete exhaustion. By going inward, you may recognize the cost to your physical and emotional health of working continuously long hours or consistently accommodating other people's needs above your own. Either action may get you kudos from external sources but both are likely distractions from your heart's light and true desire.

When the patterns of responding that have become automatic for you are brought to light, you have a chance to choose more consciously what works for you. This stage of just paying attention to reactions to the unfamiliar, to your responses to situations, ideas, and other people begins to call attention to Inner Wisdom inherent in your body's reactions.

On my own journey, I became aware of how much of my mental and emotional energy was directed externally. Once I worked to create the space that made it easier for me to be quiet than to engage my brain, I observed where the true sources of my energy were. I wrote in one of my journals:

In this process of being fully awake, fully conscious, I am more connected to Beauty and living things—with the exception of people. I am actually less connected to other people.

This was a huge observation for me because I love being with people and do derive a great deal of joy from interactions with others. It took me a relatively long time—in silence—to recognize how much of my energy was focused on helping others with whatever was affecting them at any time. I would easily divert my own energy to helping them transform their stuckness into hope and forward movement. However, my unconscious investment of energy was allowing me to indiscriminately invest my own energy in people who were not following their own paths or even doing their own work. I began to care more about their potential then they did. Because I had a great deal of energy, I could keep going, ignoring little signals in my body that gradually grew bigger until I had to notice.

Why is it that when I am not feeling well or am tired, I am also most content with just being?

As in any journey towards mastery, time and practice enable new patterns to develop. Small steps and small successes build on each other. If you are noticing more and more what gives you energy and what takes energy away, it becomes easier to seek out and support what gives you energy. Your head is delighted to do so because it would rather do what seems logical and reasonable. And it can now recognize the logic of your new choices. For example, instead of waiting until pure exhaustion or physical illness stops you from doing things that drag your energy down, you may begin to carve out space for things and people who bring you joy and say "no" to those that don't.

When I began, these three days were a disruption (albeit a sometimes pleasant one). Now I find myself less willing to explain or defend them—they are the beginning of a shift and an integral resetting of priorities, direction, and orientation to what's important in my life—and those I touch.

When you are clear about what your heart wants, it is easier for your head to evaluate the logic of potential decisions that best support where you truly want to go and who you want to be. Heart leads, head supports.

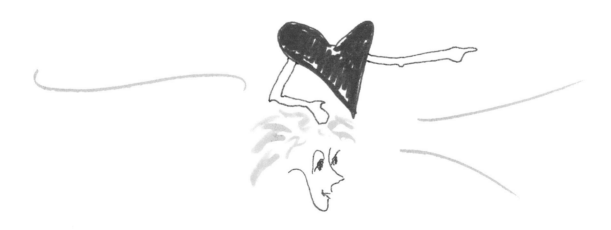

Building that awareness of head versus heart only requires that you be committed to noticing, and free from any judgments or need to do anything with what you notice. You may find it helpful to notice how you respond when you are not comfortable with what you notice. Do you find yourself trying to dismiss or otherwise get rid of any feelings of discomfort related to what you notice? When you are telling yourself that it doesn't matter that you miss a get together with friends because your team at work rescheduled a meeting without consulting your schedule, do you push the feelings of frustration aside? When an acquaintance with whom you no longer have anything in common contacts you to get together and your stomach feels sick, do you ignore the discomfort and agree to go anyway? These actions are distractions from the journey inward, and signals of the ways you give up your true Self to identify with the ego-identity you have established. In so doing, you shut down your heart's desire and Inner Wisdom.

If you do not run from or otherwise try to mask your discomfort, you create the opportunity to notice how much energy you invest in maintaining your identity. You also begin to notice how much energy it takes to keep the familiar relationships and established roles in place in order to avoid changing. Experiencing and paying attention to your feelings can help you to recognize that these old structures—old ways—are no longer serving you. It does not mean that they never served you. It only means that they do not serve you today. The time has arrived for you to choose new supports for living into your fullest potential and Highest Self.

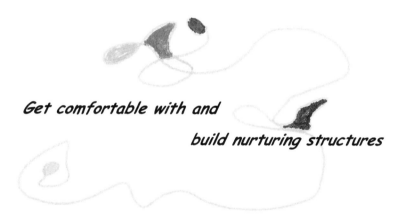

Get comfortable with and
build nurturing structures

The structures necessary to support a spiritual journey must shape the path's boundaries. This past year has challenged my boundaries, beliefs, and choices. I had to be thrust (albeit gently) out of familiar grounding to develop new eyes. It had to be different enough to challenge the status quo. The speed of life... the speed of the transformation process is what it is.

What you experience is real. When you step on a nail and you bleed, that experience is real. When you think about what happened when you stepped on the nail, you are not actually experiencing the nail piercing your skin. Whatever thoughts or emotions you conjure up by recalling the experience are only happening in your mind. Confusing your experience with your mind's interpretations of what happened slows your journey because what happens in the mind is not your true experience. It is something you make up or tell yourself about your experience.

On the journey inward, you must become conscious of what you experience in the moment and how you respond to what you experience. You must be fully present to do so—not distracting your Self with the voices in your head. Consciously choosing the physical, emotional, and thought structures that nurture your inward focus is what will help you to experience your life in the present rather than live in your head. These structures that cause you to shift your focus of attention and your behavior are structures that you consciously choose to keep your Self in the present. Anything that influences your focus of attention is a structure. It may be a belief, emotion, or physical environment that affects how you navigate your space. When you choose the thought patterns and beliefs consciously, you shift from a blind addiction to entertaining whatever thoughts occupy your mind and constrain your choices to ones that fill you with energy and joy. Thoughts and beliefs are examples of non-physical structures that either help you to be quiet and present with whatever you are experiencing or feed the powerful seduction of the mind. Once you begin to recognize what kinds of structures make it easier to experience the present moment, you are more able to live into the power of the space you are creating.

For example, imagine that you love to dance and sing. When you dance and sing, you feel free and experience absolute abandon in the moment. Your heart opens, you have lots of energy, and you fully express what is inside you. If, however, others have told you that you tend to be off-key and your dancing is stiff, you may notice that you shut off the dancing and singing when others are around. Instead of dwelling on your experience and how you feel, you dwell on the messages from other people that tell you how to experience your singing and dancing. For you to do what you love, you would need to create a space and time where you are alone, away from the judgments of others. Your space is one where you feel free to sing and dance with abandon. Such a physical and emotional space is an example of a structure that supports your going inward to experience what you love. Until you are strong enough to carry that space with you and not be affected by others' judgments, you need to create a separate physical and emotional structure—perhaps a particular room in your home or place in nature—that supports the fullest expression of your heart's desires.

Your thoughts and beliefs, conscious or unconscious, shape what you notice and how you react. Your ways of responding become forms or structures in your life. The less aware you are of them, the more insidious they are in carrying you along a path you may not even be aware you have chosen. They have become distractions from the path that serves your Highest Self, and creates ease and joy in your life. As you create the time to be quiet, with no schedule or agenda of things to do, with no expectations of anything coming out of the exercise of being quiet, you develop the capacity to notice the noise in your head, to notice how automatically you would normally respond to your head or external demands. You may even notice that you wouldn't recognize your own voice if it were trying to get your attention, because you don't know what it sounds like against the noise of other voices. The following exercise may help you to become more aware of what voices influence your behaviors and choices today.

CREATING AWARENESS OF CURRENT STRUCTURES EXERCISE

To build your capacity to go inward and hear your voice, you need to become aware of which beliefs, expectations, attitudes, and other structures currently operating in your life nurture versus distract you from going inward.

- Are you responding from your head or your heart?
- Are you aware of discomfort and other feelings as you respond?

Stay with these feelings until you can clearly see how you are nurturing versus blocking the space to connect with your heart's truth and Highest Self.

- What beliefs do you cherish that truly shape your choices and behaviors today?

- Do you have expectations about how long it should take for you to "produce" something or conclude something?

- Do you derive meaning from how many voicemail, blackberry or e-mail messages you get in a day or an hour? Why? What meaning do you attach to the number of messages?

- Is your sense of identity rooted in how you perceive that others value you? Are you sure? Check again.

- Do you find comfort in having your day scheduled? And if you say, "no" and have your days fully scheduled, check your honesty meter!

- Does feeling in control really help you to bring out your best qualities and gifts, or does it distract you from admitting how much of the real you is not being expressed or nurtured?

- What messages do you carry in your head that cause you to shut your voice down?

The purpose of these questions is to sensitize you to the voices you empower in your life and to notice whether using them to make your decisions is working for you. It may help you to record your reflections in a journal so that you can add to your insights as you notice the structures operating in your life today.

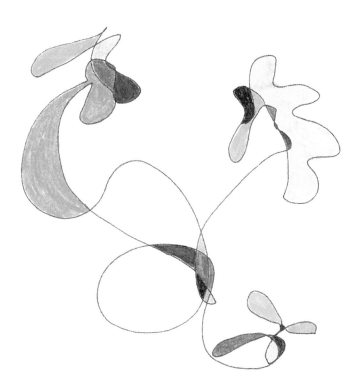

The journey to remember who you are at your core is a path to wisdom. As such it does not follow the path of planning, scheduling, and researching everything you want to know. The answers do not come from a mental process of analyzing who you are. The familiar path to becoming expert in something will not work here. It has nothing to do with figuring anything out. The path you seek is just the opposite. It is about quieting and emptying the mind, not filling it with something to do.

What becomes important is the commitment to create the silence to hear the rumblings of Inner Wisdom and the time and practice to discern your Inner Voice in the process. Towards that end, you will need to consciously choose structures—attitudes, frames of mind, favorite foods, and elements of physical comfort—that support your being in silence, that help you value your time in silence, and enable you to hear or recognize signals that direct you to more deeply know your Self. The process is not one of austerity. It is one of nurturance. What you are looking to do is to nurture the very core of who you are.

In the early stages, you may have to vigilantly guard against the tendency to distract yourself from going inward by engaging activities (structures) that you enjoy but which don't really help you go inward. For example, reading books to understand or master a concept, model, or new idea is a distraction because it engages the head rather than quieting it. Reading books written by others who are engaging the journey inward and then consciously reflecting on your own process can be very helpful. Enjoying the beauty of water or climbing a mountain may bring you a sense of peace and quiet as well, because these kinds of activities help you to be more present, and discourage your mind from distractions of the past or future. Journaling is a structure that naturally supports emptying out the clutter inside. It nurtures the process of living into the space you are creating.

> It really is the silence that creates the space to hear/receive wisdom. The discipline is to get quiet, to really value silence as Divine space. It's not so much the actual physical space, although the preparation of physical space for the express purpose of supporting silence is critical.

Coach's Tip: *An important early step is finding an environment or context that makes it easier for you to be quiet than not, easier to be present than not, and easier to notice your own responses than to respond automatically.*

For some, the space is a physical location. For others, it is found in movement such as dancing, hiking, or walking, or in any form of artistic expression such as music or visual art. All are structures that nurture the deepening of your connection with your Best Self. There is no right or wrong here; there is only what works for your Best Self.

What you are building is emotional space that allows you to expand into more of your essence. It is time for you to move beyond the box that has become your life. You might find it helpful to think of the exercise as building an extension on your home. In the process, you are determining what you want in the space to nurture your Best Self. If you like to look out the window and listen to the rain on the roof, what kind of structures—physical, emotional or thought—will you create to ensure that you provide such an opportunity for your Self? Nurture your heart's desire, not the mind's distraction of judging what you "should" want.

> It was all a nesting instinct to create the space to receive wisdom. So simple and so clear. The activities themselves are not so critical but the presence, enjoyment, following intuition lead to where all needs to be. Conscious attention to (1) being present (2) truth about heart's desire—

and whether anything in either the activity or orientation to it (being) needs to be modified are what's required.

As you experiment with what kinds of structures feel nurturing and make going inward easier, you may find in the beginning that the unconscious power of your mind supports the tendency to keep your usual ways of structuring your time, changing only the activities that fill the space. For example, if you have a tendency to be productive and get a lot of things done in a day, when you are trying to be quiet, you may schedule activities that you think of as nurturing, such as a long walk or an hour to draw. You are actually repeating your usual structured day, where you know what you are going to do next. You are filling any quiet or stillness with some of the treats you usually deny your Self. That may be fine to get you started, but stay attuned to your body's response to how the old scheduled structure feels. In time, you will be more present to how that structure affects you. You will find that pre-planning your days actually makes you less present or free to engage the experience that moves you in the moment. Follow the direction of what your heart wants as you become more and more aware of how current structures interfere with your heart's desires.

We get so enamored of and attached to how the space must look and feel that we go beyond principles to detailed rules/expectations. These detailed expectations become forms that actually constrain access to Wisdom/Truth. We hold onto human expectation and stop creating a welcome field for Divine expression.

The first thing to do when you recognize this pattern is to learn how to get a kick out of your Self! Be grateful for the ability to recognize your need to structure the day. Then learn to ask your Self what would really delight you in the time you have set aside. In time, you will find that no set schedule nurtures your heart's desire. What your heart may actually want at a particular moment is to do nothing. Then do that and notice what it feels like.

You are developing the capacity to ask your Self what you really want in that moment and follow whatever delights your Highest Self. The "doing" will go down and noticing your "being"—how you feel physically and emotionally, and the qualities elicited in you—will go up. You are developing your own space and trusting what happens in each moment to help you consciously recognize what will support that silence. You are also beginning to follow inner direction by allowing your Self not only to do nothing, but also to delight in doing nothing.

If I had been given a framework, I would not have to have been so aware. I could have followed it unconsciously—as one follows a well-laid path. It's not that I wouldn't have paid attention to new pieces along the trail. It's more that that's all I would have paid attention to—and for only so long as it took me to get from point A to point B.

We often only stop to notice what is working and what isn't when we are literally stopped in our tracks from doing what we have always done in the way we have always done it. Creating a nurturing space where you feel safe and able to open your eyes to what might be seen anew is what will allow you to go deeper into the silence and to welcome the unfamiliar without fear. You experience a genuine openness to discovery. And that's a space to which you will want to return, because it nurtures you at a very deep level. It is tranquil and exhilarating all at once.

In the early part of going inward—because it is so foreign for so many of us in any kind of sustained way in our lives—the process of becoming aware of unconscious patterns must be paramount. Noticing what's familiar and noticing the tendency to want to fit each new experience into a labeled category that gives it familiar place and meaning is natural. But remember, the goal here is not to recreate what is already familiar or comfortable. It is to discover how ingrained your patterns and frameworks for structuring your life have become. It's a little like being a fish in a pond and awakening to the realization that you are living in the water! You don't see the environment you live in unless you consciously step back and get some perspective on where you are. What may help is to develop a new language for describing the experience that will help you to see it differently.

> *Metaphor is a tremendously powerful bridge language, providing some grounding for making meaning of new experiences—outside the realm of current ways of thinking and conscious knowing. It provides a way to picture, imagine, connect something in a way that holds the door open to accept/validate the new experience and hold the space/frame to integrate a new perspective.*

The metaphor of a garden served my own process because I could grasp that for several months after making a commitment to being alone in silence—but not without chocolate or walks along the ocean— something was happening, even though I might not actually see any changes. I could understand that by setting aside the time and trusting the process, I was essentially clearing the ground and planting the seeds. Even though it would be a long winter before I saw anything sprout, I could understand that a lot was growing below the surface. My choices were nurturing the fertile ground that would be receptive to rich discovery. Recognition of my own voice was being cultivated every time that I set aside time, made a conscious commitment to creating space to go inward, and freed myself of expectations that I would have anything to "report" at the end of the time I had set aside. You may find other metaphors useful, as well, to describe and provide perspective on your own inward process.

Coach's Tip: Consider using a visual picture or metaphor to frame the process of creating space to go inward—in-dwelling—in a way that eases your mind and helps you stay with the process until you can consciously know how much you yearn for that space in your life!

Once you have created the space in your life, pay attention to how it is serving you. When what you need is no longer served by the space or support structures you have created, it is time to change the structures. Nearly three years to the month of the conversation that had sparked my decision to create space for what needed to happen in my life, I became aware that I did not need to set aside three days each month. Old patterns that no longer worked for me had become clearer and I was much more connected to my body signals and intuition. I recognized that it was time to move on in a way that I would carry my space with me in my "regular life." I wrote in my journal:

> *I can release the three days. They constituted a structure and it has served its purpose. I'm discarding that shell for a new one. It was foreign enough to force me to stop and pay attention. And it was not so overwhelming as to discourage me.*

Until you begin to create the space in your life to go inward, you may find that you unconsciously hold on tightly to familiar structures—patterns of behavior, ways of getting results—without remembering why you put them in place initially. As a result, you may devote a great deal of energy to maintaining the structures long after they have outlived their usefulness. The goal of creating space for me to become more conscious of who I am being and what serves my Highest Self required three days of silence because I needed something to shock me out of my old routines. As I developed a stronger relationship with my own wisdom and what brings me joy, I also learned to value preserving the space in my life to remain conscious. The initial structure of three days is no longer the most effective way for me to do my work in the world. I have built new structures that are shorter and more frequent to support my connection with Highest Self as I continue on my path. As you build new nurturing structures for wherever you are on your journey, stay open to recognizing when you are using energy to feed a structure that no longer serves your process of focusing inward.

In the in-dwelling process, the first step we have been exploring is how to *create the space to go inward.* The next phase or step in the journey back Home is to:

Shine the Light on Unconscious Patterns and Behaviors

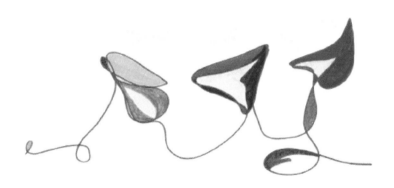

Now that you have created the space in which to be quiet, you are ready to see what wants growth and what you are growing that you do not want to grow. This is a time of absolute honesty and rigorous attachment to shining light on all you see. Teaching your mind that there is nothing you will see that you cannot address in a way that brings out the very best in you is important. Otherwise, you may be tempted to duck out of seeing where you are putting your energy today that may not be serving your Highest Self at all. This is an opportunity to get your eyes and ears calibrated for truth-telling. If you were going on a safari at night and wanted to spot animals camouflaged in the bush, you would need bright lights to discern them from their surroundings. The exact same thing is true here. You are embarking on an adventure into some hidden corners of your mind and life to discover what is real and what is just a façade that you are unconsciously supporting.

The unconscious façade is nothing more than the ego-identity that you have built to be successful in the world, please others, or gain some kind of external validation. The identity in which you have cloaked your Self no longer fits. Before you discard it, you will need to be very clear about exactly what it is that no longer suits you. Compassionately discern —that means be gentle with your Self —what aspects of your life are not supporting your Best Self and without judging or criticizing, discard them. The process is one of shining the light, noticing and naming what you see as distractions from being your Highest Self, and then walking away.

Notice and name distractions—and move on

When you shine a light on the choice to either use your energy to maintain an identity that gets you outside validation or to experience your own light, the cost-benefit ratio of your decision becomes clearer. The fears associated with really seeing who you are without reference to titles, roles, and positions in the physical world melt away as curiosity about how you got to where you are claim your attention. The desire to know whether you are hanging onto an identity, relationship, or behavior out of fear, guilt, or doubt is stronger than actually continuing to hold on. You are more tied to knowing the truth than to the comfort of maintaining the status quo. Such clear intention to ferret out what is real and hear your Inner Voice creates a sense of curiosity, and a lack of judgment or fear about what might happen. You are hooked on the journey—not the destination.

The context is set for you to become an astute observer of your Self in action. Your ability to notice what gets your attention expands. You become aware that what you need to do is first to *notice,* and then *name* what games your mind plays. You then also notice and name what distractions from the past or anticipated future hold sway over whatever you are experiencing at that moment. Once you notice and name, moving on is much easier. The unconscious hooks to ego-identity are loosening. The skids are greased for you to become more conscious and more able to move in light, rather than darkness, fear, or pain. You are more open to hearing the Wisdom within you. You more easily recognize the voices of others playing in your head as they offer their uninvited perspectives on the way things are or should be as outside voices, not necessarily your own truth. Shining a light on these unconscious voices means paying attention to the voices in your head to the point where you can discern which ones ring true and which ones don't ring true for the person you choose to be. This process requires a vigilant watching of the mind in action, as if it were a separate entity from your Self.

> *It's tricky to silence the wily mind. Feeling at peace and quiet for a longer period of time than you may usually experience often invites the mind or time clock to create anxiety or daydreams about unresolved issues or future fears. These distractions play out like an evening at the theatre. At some time during the "performance," you will awaken to the fact that you have been daydreaming, effectively tricked by the mind into leaving the state of calm and quiet that is the present and preoccupying yourself with games of the mind.*

If you are committed to staying in the present, you will recognize the mind's attempts to distract you and stop it. If your commitment to being present is strong enough, it is possible to consciously let the mind know that you are not budging, and that you are continuing to evaluate which of the voices competing for your attention feels true to your heart. You create the space to hear your own truth. In the moment it takes to choose to stop the less-than-conscious mind from dictating behavior, you are beginning to recognize the mind's games and tactics. Often messages are darting around in your head, attempting to get you back "on track," a disguise for returning to ego-identity and the status quo. These voices or messages may sound something like: "I don't have time for this." "This is taking too long." "This is ridiculous." "They're going to think I'm crazy." "Am I crazy?"

Without patience, focus, and a commitment to the in-dwelling process, you may find it easier and eminently more fascinating to be distracted by the wanderings and games of the mind to stay in control, rather than to experience and feel what is happening at the moment. Leaning into discomfort or uncertainty and trusting the heart is not a natural path for many of us. But during critical stages in life—transitions—pressure to listen to your heart increases and you become more aware of the value of doing so.

Mid-life is one example. It often brings with it a newfound urgency to discern what is important to us and what we want in the second half of life. For many, the recognition that life as we know it is probably half over presents a stark message that each choice really matters. It always has, but now we are more prepared to listen because it is harder to deny a message about time passing and our lives meaning something when the big 40, 50, or 60 shows up. For some, this realization will promote immediate denial and the re-creation of earlier patterns such as jumping into relationships with significantly younger partners to avoid feeling old or buying the newest toy or gadget that supports our view of ourselves as young and vital. The real opportunity is to step back, notice what is going on, and honestly assess what feels real and true. You will find that you need stillness for the light to clearly separate truth from façade, to reconnect you with your passions and neglected loves. It is a time to defy conventional wisdom and develop the strength of voice that resonates with what your heart has been trying to tell you for years.

TRUTH-TELLING EXERCISE

This exercise will help you to feel more comfortable shining light on your fears and limiting beliefs, rather than being distracted by them. It may take practice. Be patient with yourself.

As you answer the questions below, if you experience any pangs of fear, doubt, guilt, or discomfort, sit with those feelings. Look them squarely in the eye until you understand what meaning you assign to the answer you gave to the question. Pay attention to what the voice in your head is saying.

- Whose voice is it?

- Where have you heard those words before?

Then ask yourself what the worst case is if you do not listen to that voice. You can more truthfully recognize that the reality of the worst-case scenario is not as you have conjured it up and judged it in your head. Notice your reaction, name it, and stay with it until you are ready to let it go.

- When does the way you do your job bring out the Best in you? When does it not?

- Are you where you want to be in your life?

- Which of your relationships are fulfilling? Which ones are not?

- Do you have a sense of making a difference with your life? When?

- What brings you joy?

- What fuels your passion?

- Do you recognize your passion amidst the activities in your life?

- Do you see yourself and your desires in the big picture of your life or are you invisible in order to focus on all whom you (nobly) serve?

- Are your choices serving your Highest Self? Usually? Often? Seldom? Never?

Keep shining the light on the answers to these questions. This activity can be immensely liberating and much more comforting in the long run than self-medicating through some pattern of distraction or escape.

Much to the chagrin of whole generations who have happily entrusted their choices to others, no outside expert can answer these questions for you better than your heart can. It is time to sit back and watch your Self and the choices you make. It is time to notice and name the choices, patterns, and ruts that have become you. And it is critical that you do so with a sense of discovery and humor rather than judgment.

Your awareness of conformity as a means of control within society increases when you pay attention to the messages in your head that you willingly, and sometimes blindly, obey. Noticing the thinking that shapes how you respond to a situation can be tremendously powerful in and of itself, even if you don't initially change your responses. When you continue to focus your attention on both the messages and how you respond to them, you take control of your life back from your unconscious mind. You are becoming a more active player in your own life simply by watching and reflecting on your choices and responses.

As you naturally observe your Self, you will find it easier to name what you see and not judge yourself harshly for past choices. You become more focused on being honest with your Self for who you choose to be today. The past disappears from focus. Worrying about who you become in the future is held up to the light for what it is—a mind game to distract you from experiencing your Self in the present. When you keep the focus on the present, you notice what is happening, name it without judging, and move on to the next present moment. You become aware that the fun is in choosing who you are in each present moment and in seeing how you actually get there—no judging, just watching and experiencing.

It is natural when learning something new to draw strong boundaries between the old way and the new. This black and white distinction highlights the differences and makes it easier not to hide from new learnings and observations. For example, rather than seeing that you are "mostly" or "somewhat" honest in a relationship, you begin to look more closely at when you are honest and when it is easier for you to be less than honest with your feelings and thoughts. You begin to look more closely at the details, such as with whom you are more honest. You can see more clearly with whom you are your Best Self and who or what circumstances bring out the worst in you.

Coach's Tip: Developing a fierce vigilance for truth allows you to not only notice the actions and patterns you choose but to also name them, without any need to judge yourself for past actions.

Truth becomes critically important and tremendously freeing. You become more able to name and assess whether what you recognize to be happening is in service of your highest purpose and Best Self or not. The level of questioning intensifies. You hold yourself accountable to your Highest Self, to all that is best in you to answer why you are not choosing to manifest those qualities and gifts. The journey inward continues and your ability to separate what is real from illusion is accelerated. It is a time of increased self-confidence and it is not self sustaining. You have to stay alert because the mind is not giving up! It has been in charge for a number of years, perhaps decades, and it is not happy to have a worthy competitor—the heart—getting more attention and power.

With continued commitment to becoming more conscious and to stepping into your highest potential, you can reassure the mind that it has a critical role to play. The role is different, but no less powerful. Rather than lead, it is charged with enabling you to make real the desires of your heart, to help you manifest your Best Self and highest potential. In order to get there, you have to prepare yourself to be willing to abandon everything that stands in your way, to change any relationship that does not foster your highest potential. You need to sit with this thought a minute, until you feel its truth.

> *There's a major cycle/phase of emptying out, clearing away. It's a clearing of weeds that have grown, overgrowth of plants that are crowding out the Beauty of the well-tended garden. The clearing and what needs to grow become paramount. Then it's easier to design conscious structures that keep human choices more aligned with Divine wisdom and the power of the path/ process is more sustainable (with care and feeding).*

Once the pattern of noticing without judging and then naming the experience without adding meaning is ingrained, letting go and moving on are natural. The awareness of the burden of continuing to foster old patterns so that others will not become uncomfortable, angry, or reject you, is a wake-up call to choose what supports your Highest Self. You can more easily choose not to carry the burden of the old patterns because the cost of doing so to your Best Self is clear. You begin to recognize the sources of dis-ease in your life and choose not to hide from your role in creating them through your choices to deny your heart and then convince your Self you had no choice.

The light is now shining on the cost of decisions made from cowardice. The patterns of hiding from choices you know you need to make, regardless of how insignificant or how big, are exposed for what they are. And the freedom to create your life from this very moment forward shines through. It doesn't mean that the road is always easy—especially when you unconsciously resist your truth or are addicted to distractions you are not prepared to recognize. It does mean that everyone has the power to step into his or her highest potential and walk more in light than in darkness. It is about making conscious choices that serve your Best Self, and in turn all you love most.

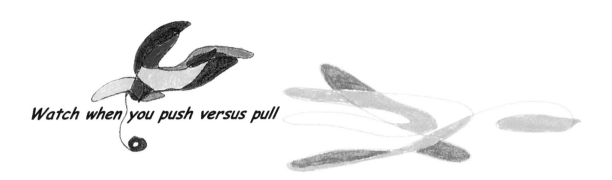

Watch when you push versus pull

A dilemma we encounter on this journey inward is how much to push versus how much to wait patiently until something unfolds or presents itself. There is no easy answer, but there is wisdom to be found within each of us about when to use each approach. The context of our individual choices and backgrounds makes stating a general rule of waiting versus pushing impractical, if not misleading. But when the journey becomes too difficult, when your focus shifts from what you deeply desire to a focus on timing—believing that something you want isn't happening fast enough—you're probably pushing too hard and not being quiet enough to listen. There's a pretty good chance that at moments like these you have become less conscious of your own process and more inclined to follow the time impositions of the mind. These would not be your more enlightened moments!

> *...we tend to give all the power to the result when the real power is the process. My three days are a magical time, yielding tremendous abundance but not in the form, way, or time frame I tend to expect...At about the point I think I need to push something, I tend to develop an "oh well, resignation" or abandon. It's at that point that I'm open to creating, to receiving something new.*

The process of recognizing when to push or pull is a journey towards mastery—the mastery of clear intention and cultivated silence to recognize and receive the wisdom that emerges. We often do not recognize the help that is there for each of us on our paths. Most of the confusion occurs when you are not absolutely clear about what you ultimately want. You then confuse how you get there with what you want. If your ego is invested in how you achieve what you want, you are likely to push too hard and miss clues for how to have what you want with ease. For example, if you want a promotion and you believe the way to be promoted is to have the support of one particular manager, you are likely to push that manager in ways that don't allow your Highest Self to be present. At the same time, a peer may offer to position you for the very same promotion but you don't recognize the help being sent your way because you either view the peer as a competitor or not in a position to help you. You are too busy pushing your agenda to stand back silently and observe that an alternate approach, such as accepting your peer's help, could get you what you want with less effort.

Likewise, if you are not particularly clear about what you want, you may not push hard enough to attract opportunities you would like to have. If you would like to be considered for a new position, but are not clear about what skills you want to enhance or why you might want a new position, others won't know how to help you make the necessary connections to identify and access relevant opportunities. More is written about when to effectively push versus pull later in the book under the section on Grace. What is critical here is to develop the practice of consciously shining the light on times in your life where you feel tired or defeated, perhaps pushing against someone or something and times when you get what you want with ease.

OBSERVING EXERCISE

Stand back and observe your behaviors. Remove yourself from any emotional reaction and instead truly observe your behaviors, as you answer the questions that follow:

- Are you pushing or pulling? Are you forcing anything?

- What results are you getting from whichever route you are taking?

- Are you reconnecting with your Best Self and getting what you want?

- Do you like who you are becoming in the situation you are observing?

- Are you conscious of your choices and what motivates them in the situation?

- Are your choices supporting your heart's desires and the Best in you?

Don't judge. Just shine the light and develop the capacity to see what results you are getting from your choices. Keep looking until you can see the relationship among your choices, your Highest Self, and the situations you find yourself attracting. For those situations where you are not getting what you want with ease, where you feel you are pushing and nothing is happening, look closely at whether there were clues you might have overlooked about how to achieve your heart's desire.

Being able to create the quiet and non-judging mind that does not drive or push decisions may be new for you. Unlearning the old and mastering the new takes conscious focus and discipline. Meditation is one of the most accessible ways of disciplining the mind to sit quietly while Wisdom presents itself.

Meditate to expand consciousness

When I was first directed to get quiet, I was also advised to meditate. I suspect many of you may be far more experienced at what meditation means and feels like than I was. I read books and bought tapes to figure out what meditation was. I built up expectations about how it would feel, how long it should take, and what the results would be. I waited for these things to happen. Most didn't. But the process was fun—in retrospect. I did learn to let go of my expectations and the need to figure out the "right way." When I finally got my head out of the way, I learned what a rich resource meditation can be for reconnecting with my heart and Inner Wisdom.

In the early days I learned to congratulate myself if, on a walk, my mind could be quiet for up to thirty seconds. I did that for many walks! As time progressed, and I finally let go of how I thought meditation should feel and how it would work, I gradually increased the time my mind was quiet and became acutely aware of how preoccupied my mind was with work or other concerns. I couldn't fathom valuing a quiet mind. I had to learn to wait **with**—not **for**—the quiet. I continued to wonder what good a quiet mind would be. But I stayed with it and found out. I know for certain that if *I* could learn to slow down and really experience the benefits of expanding my consciousness through meditation, then anyone who chooses to do the same can do it.

One of the most helpful pieces of information to remember about meditation is that it does not need to be complicated. At the most basic level, meditation only means quieting the mind. It may take any of a number of forms. You do not need to be sitting in lotus position chanting a mantra to meditate, although many do. I found that walking meditations work best for me. Walking meditation simply means that I was moving while quieting my mind, and that I was using the rhythm of movement and the changing surroundings to help me get more present. I focused on the temperature, the sounds around me, the sky, how the ground felt, and whatever I passed on my walk to keep me present. I learned how to be quiet and present. I could still make necessary adjustments—like getting out of the way of approaching cars or people—to stay upright! I learned soft vision, where I would focus on everything and nothing specific at the same time to keep me present and able to avoid potholes and fallen branches on my path. Even if thoughts would occupy my mind, I would become aware of them and choose to shift my attention to watching my mind, experiencing my surroundings, or focusing on my breathing.

For me, the goal of meditative practice is to create the conditions where my mind goes beyond traditional thinking to a place of quiet. It is peacefully exhilarating. The practice of going beyond noticing physical objects to that space where everything is both vibrantly alive and still is tremendously peaceful. For those of you who have to give your mind a goal in order to stay engaged, creating a still and quiet mind is the goal.

> *... a knowing comes over me—and it defies description...a whole new perspective on everything appears—in one felt swoop. This is not a "slow reveal" of one step at a time. Suddenly the veil is lifted and the whole is clear—all at once. It's immense in its spaciousness.*

There are many different techniques and tools to help you meditate and expand your consciousness. Some offer the absolute opposite advice of that offered by others. Some recommend you repeat a prayer, phrase, or expression continuously. Others recommend you pay absolute attention to all sounds going on around you at once to develop presence and mindfulness. Still others recommend that you get quiet and focus on your breath until that is all you notice. There is no right or wrong method. Whatever helps you to become more conscious of being present and also quiets your mind is an approach that works for you. The Goldilocks approach works just fine—sample each bowl of porridge until you choose the one that is just right for you.

The good news is that you can approach meditation as you might approach any new activity—playfully. Get a kick out of how often your mind tries to interrupt. Some people actually put their minds in "time out" by noticing whenever a stray thought arrives. When they recognize the uninvited visitor, they promptly escort it to a "room" of their favorite color, as in, "How nice of you to visit. She's not available right now, but if you'd like to wait in the blue room, she'll back in a half hour." If you tend to be intense, you'll need to relax by explicitly telling yourself how long you are going to be meditating so that you can keep reminding yourself—in much the same way as you might speak to a child who interrupts you to get your attention—that time is not up and you are not ending any earlier than planned.

A disciplined mind can be put in check. An undisciplined mind runs amok like an out-of-control child demanding attention.

There are many books on meditation that you may find helpful. The point here is to strongly encourage you to select a venue that is natural for you and keep practicing, as you would with any new sport, musical instrument, or activity you seek to master. If you like the outdoors, go there. The physical space in which you meditate must be soothing and calming for you, because the physical environment helps you create the emotional environment that makes it easier to get quiet and simply be open to what happens. It doesn't have to be any more complicated than that. The following exercise may help you get started.

BEGINNING MEDITATION EXERCISE (STATIONARY)

Plan for this time to be nurturing and peaceful by choosing a physical environment that is quiet and where you will not be disturbed. Put on music that has no clear beat or rhythm (Native American flute music or Tibetan bowls, for example) and no words (unless you have a meditation CD that uses a repetitive chant, mantra, or guided visualization).

- Sit upright on a chair that supports your back.

- Uncross your arms and legs and plant your feet firmly on the floor.

- Either close your eyes or focus your gaze on something that does not move.

- Begin by imagining that there are roots coming from the bottom of your feet that go all the way to the center of the earth.

- Stay focused on these roots as you begin to focus on your breath.

- Imagine that, with each breath in you are breathing in wisdom and energy.

- With each exhale, you are releasing through the roots in the soles of your feet all the stress and tension you carry.

- Repeat this breathing until you feel relaxed.

- When you feel no more tension, pay attention to the quiet or the music around you as you continue to breathe in energy and wisdom. Exhale any thoughts that pop into your mind.

- Keep doing this until your mind is quiet.

Do this exercise any time you want to release stress. It can take anywhere from a few minutes to as long as you find it helpful.

For those of you who prefer to be moving, you may find a walking meditation easier to integrate into your activities. The opportunity to be outdoors, experiencing all of the beauty of nature gives many people a very natural way to slow the mind and become more present. Consider the following walking meditation exercise as a way to begin.

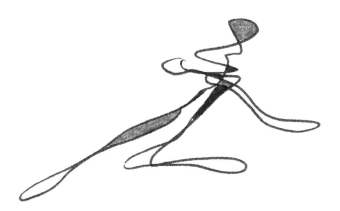

BEGINNING MEDITATION EXERCISE (WALKING)

Unlike the stationary meditation exercise, this exercise is about developing "soft vision." This means that you will be alert to your surroundings while not focusing intensely on any specific entities you may encounter. For people who have trouble sitting still, walking meditation is a much more natural way to learn to quiet your mind, because you are continuously in motion.

- Choose an environment where you will encounter as few people as possible and keep your eyes open! Now you are ready to begin.

- Imagine that there is a magnet under the ground that is connected to the bottom of your feet or shoes.

- Imagine that the magnet attached to each foot is a large open-ended cylinder that is also attached to the center of the earth. Each magnetic cylinder is hidden beneath the surface of the earth and moves with you wherever you go. The cylinders are attached to and carry the wisdom and energy of life itself within them.

- Take your hands out of your pockets and allow them to move freely as you walk. Notice your posture and carry yourself upright.

- As you take each step, pay attention to the feel of the ground beneath your feet.

- Listen to the sounds around you.

- Pay attention to all you see.

- Now, as you pay attention to your senses, begin to focus on your breath.

- Imagine that with each breath in you are breathing in wisdom and energy.

- With each exhale you are releasing all the stress and tension you carry through the bottom of your feet into the cylinder.

- Notice any thoughts that pop into your head and release them through your feet, allowing the magnetic force to draw them away and leave you with a quiet mind.

- Continue to pay attention to the sounds, sights, and sensations you experience as you walk, while remaining conscious of your breath.

- If you lose focus on your breath and then notice that your mind is preoccupied with thoughts, simply return focus to your breath again. No judgment. Just keep focusing on your senses as you walk.

- You may notice that the pace of both your walking and breathing has slowed. Simply enjoy what happens.

These and other meditation exercises will help you to discipline your mind, become more conscious, and reconnect with your heart. You may also find that they naturally foster a slower, quieter, and clearer frame of mind that helps you to remain more alert and creative in other activities that follow.

Your ability to reconnect with the highest and best in you depends on your willingness to create space and quiet in your life, your willingness to practice in-dwelling. Once you have *created space* and developed your capacity to *shine light on unconscious patterns and behaviors*, it is time to attune your listening and hearing. The sheer volume of noise in your life, whether physical sounds of media and the external world or the constant yammering of voices in your head, can make it difficult for you to both recognize and hear the important messages of your heart. That ability to sift through the noise to uncover the wisdom is the last major step of in-dwelling. It is time for you to hone your ability to:

Discern Inner Wisdom from Noise

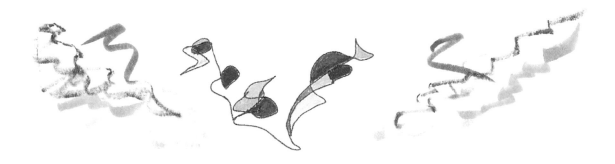

In the context of everyday noise you may not be attuned to the inspired truth that your heart carries when you are fully present and conscious. That inspired truth is a kind of cellular knowing that points you towards the path of purpose, ease, and joy. It is Inner Wisdom and it is easily accessible to all who choose to live from the heart. When you have developed some kind of disciplined practice for creating space to be quiet and increased ability to shine light on your unconscious patterns and behaviors, you are ready to focus your attention on hearing that Inner Wisdom. To do so, you will need to incorporate a deep desire to really hear the Wisdom carried through a variety of channels, and especially embedded in your intuition, into your conscious intentions. This last step of in-dwelling—movement towards Home on the Soul Grid—is about preparing the soil to receive the seeds of Wisdom that grow your magnificent garden. These are the seeds that nurture and celebrate the fullest expression of your Highest Self. The process of discerning Inner Wisdom from noise begins with focused intention to really listen for Wisdom in all sorts of forms and contexts.

Listen attentively _for_ Inner Wisdom

When you focus on listening **_for_** someone or something to appear, you will find that you can listen beyond the usual noise and distractions. When you are listening **_for_**, it is about clear intention. If you are expecting someone to arrive, you may be listening for any indication of his or her arrival—a car engine, footstep, key in the door, or sound of a voice. Initially, you may find that you are listening **_to_** only certain kinds of messages, because you imagine that those are the ways in which Wisdom will appear.

Imagine that you are celebrating a good friend's recent promotion. Your friend is describing how he learned of his promotion. You are listening **_to_** his words, paying attention to his story. If you also recognize your intention to celebrate his success and support him in feeling good about his achievements, you will find that you are able to listen to what he is not saying, as well. You can do this because your body will help you listen **_for_** ways to celebrate and support him. You may pick up on his fear that he is not as good as his boss thinks he is. You will have a sense of where he is hesitating. If you are conscious of messages suggesting how to respond or what to say to fulfill your intention to celebrate and support his success, you will know when to intervene to remind him of his strengths and support his confidence. You will be able to access Wisdom that helps you achieve your intention with ease. Gradually, with continued practice, you will recognize how you receive intuitive messages and be able to access and use this Inner Voice—Wisdom—in the moment.

Intuition is the inner spiritual voice of knowing that sees beyond immediate human reasoning and demands to reveal what's called for. And it becomes a calling, an urging even, to pay attention. It's a calling Home—a time to unwind, become consciously aware…It's an inspired voice and an inspired calling. As such it may not use a language we're used to listening to to get our attention.

The Inner Voice of Wisdom does not lie. The mind may. The Inner Voice is not emotionally tied to one particular outcome or another. The mind usually is. The Inner Voice often prompts an immediate signaling of something that would protect you from harm or move you to greater heights. The Inner Voice moves with compassion and without judgment. It is the voice of the heart, the voice of the Soul, and the Wisdom that is often recognized as intuition. Here is how it works:

You may have felt called to take a particular job at a point in time or to help someone whom you didn't know well for reasons you couldn't articulate, only to find that something you learned or someone you met through that activity became crucial to a next step in your own life. That's how intuition works. It isn't always direct in the rational mind's definition of directness. But it is wonderfully efficient at supporting your Highest Self and life path, if you are willing to entertain its invitation.

Hearing the wisdom of intuition and following that wisdom are two different things. But one thing is for sure—if you cannot or will not hear the Inner Voice, you are certainly not inclined to follow it! You may be signaled by your body that you are pushing too hard, denying your Self nurturance, not setting clear boundaries in your relationships, burying your voice, and acting as though you have a lock on what is right and just. If you don't recognize the signals about what these behaviors are costing you, you will not be inclined to address the signaled need to change. It is this lack of attunement to Wisdom's voice that leads many to only change when they are faced with so much drama, darkness, and pain in their lives that they have to listen if they want to survive. Does this path sound familiar to you? It doesn't have to be this way.

Intuition is accessible to everyone and accessing it is like playing the piano or exercising a new muscle. The more you do it, the more natural it becomes. Everyone is born with access to Inner Wisdom. Some work harder to deny it. Children often connect with it very easily, until socialized out of listening to their Inner Voice and directed to play by society's rules for rewards and acceptance. In fact, children are often carriers of the precise wisdom messages that we have avoided hearing from a variety of sources. We commonly react to wisdom spoken by a child by proclaiming, "out of the mouths of babes" when a child speaks a truth immediately recognized but not spoken by adults.

Intuition is nothing to be feared. The wisdom embedded in what we call intuition is in service of our Highest Self. What could be scary about that? Unless you have decided that you know better than a Supreme Source of Wisdom what is best for you and how to unleash your highest potential, listening can only create the opportunity to move you closer to joy and Highest Self. However, because Inner Wisdom does not lie and because it is not attached to unhealthy relationships you may be engaging today, the messages may be difficult to hear. If you are attached to hearing a particular message, then you are not listening *for* Wisdom and intuition simply cannot get through. The line is busy and intuition doesn't compete to be heard in that moment. It may choose to call back though, so you could have another chance!

Hearing the Divine, the Inner Voice seems a process of becoming conscious of all the other voices holding sway. Making the unconscious underlying voices conscious exposes the ego's role of social expectations on conduct and beliefs. Unwinding that part of the pattern by making it more explicit, visible, conscious opens the possibility of hearing the heart (Inner) voice. The Soul's imperative to meet in Silence can be honored because now the other voices, with light shining on them, can be put in perspective.

Unless you have cultivated a soil receptive to different forms of messages by separating what you want in your heart from how your head tells you to go about getting what you want, you may not recognize the help in the form it arrives. How many times have you rejected wisdom presented to you about how to handle a particular situation or life choice because you did not recognize it in the form it was presented to you or because the advice came from someone who didn't fit your expectations of a wise person or "qualified" expert? I once passed up a perfect opportunity on my path for exactly this reason.

I had been looking for a parking place, a premium property in the town where I lived. One came available in the form of a wonderful studio apartment around the corner from my home. Not only would I have gotten the parking place I needed, I would have found the perfect art studio. But I still wasn't sure whether to buy the property because I was listening to my head's doubts about whether I really needed the apartment. When I went to sleep that night I asked myself what to do. When I awoke the next morning, the words of a song were playing in my head. They were, " one in a million, chance of a lifetime." I chuckled and even told a good friend about the song lyrics that seemed to answer my question. I still did not listen to my heart's excitement about the studio. I allowed my head to get in the way of my heart's message. I asked someone I considered more knowledgeable about whether I should buy the property. His advice was not to do so. I followed his advice. The apartment sold.

A year later, another apartment the same size with a parking space opened in the same building. I jumped at it. Only this time, in order to buy the apartment I wanted, I had to pay 25% more to get it! So, although I did eventually get the opportunity to do what would serve my path, it cost me more, because I did not listen to my Inner Voice when it first tried to get my attention. That wonderful studio ended up being one of the places where I found solace to do my in-dwelling. How could I have known at the time that I would need a space that was quiet and solitary? Wisdom tried to tap me on the shoulder and I refused it entry because I allowed my head to judge the form in which it came. Developing the conscious intention to listen *for* Wisdom allows you to be more alert to the help when it arrives and less inclined to judge the form in which it appears by conventional standards. Wisdom is not about convention!

To develop your own capacity to recognize Wisdom, consider the following exercise:

STRETCHING EXERCISE

To go beyond your usual boundaries of comfort, consider paying attention to times in your life when you feel you are asking for help and getting no response. In those moments where you feel abandoned or unheard, notice such things as:

• What song lyrics are playing in your head, or on the radio/sound system?

• What part of your body is signaling any kind of discomfort?

• What ideas pop into your head from "nowhere" or come from unlikely sources, such as children or animals?

Now notice how often you dismiss or refuse entry to any of these potential aids because you judge them unworthy of serious consideration. *Is it that you are so tied to how the help must come that you do not recognize it when it arrives in a different form?* Consider giving your Self the opportunity to listen to or consider potential help hidden in these, or other forms and just remain open to what happens. You may find that you do not need to push much; you only need to pull towards you what is already there to help you.

As you can see, discerning Wisdom requires conscious intention and openness to hearing the messages. It is much easier to recognize Inner Wisdom when you have created the physical, emotional, and mental space to hear it. When you are willing to slow your mind and more deliberately focus your intention, you will find it easier to recognize where the voices of "conventional wisdom" distract you from your Inner Voice. To accelerate your connection with Wisdom, make sure to find the time and space to explore and nurture your creativity.

Nurture creative self expression

Reconnecting with your unique voice of creative expression helps create the space for Wisdom to appear because you are more directly connected with what you love, with what makes you smile. Contrary to what you have been told—or tell yourself—you are creative. All humans are. The form of creativity may vary—making a special meal, arranging a home, listening to music, dancing, sculpting, quilting, or whatever inspires you to quiet the voices inside and create. The form of creative expression that inspires or warms your heart is yours to discover. Just know that it is there—maybe buried under a world of perceived responsibilities and obligations—but there. So, take the time to find it because it will attune you to your Inner Voice, your Highest Self.

The poet uses words to express the experience—co-creates with the words and the Spirit behind them. A sculptor waits to find out what the wood/stone wants to be and listens to the voices to know how to proceed. The artist's imperative is to express. To express means there's an experience to be expressed. Experiencing the ordinary and expressing what's extraordinary gets closer to real faith and beauty.

Whatever language of creativity transports you from dismissing an inkling or sense as unimportant or ordinary to recognizing its beauty and wisdom, pay attention to that form of creativity. It is an access point to Inner Wisdom and your Highest Self. You will know it when you stop to recognize when you feel both at peace and energized, when time stands still and you are totally present in whatever you are doing. Be careful not to judge creativity by society's measures. Any activity that allows you to express what is in your heart, whether you know what it is in advance or whether you discover your heart's message in performing the activity, is a form of creativity that allows you to express what is held inside of you. Remember that it is an inside-out process. You are not putting information in; you are finding a means of drawing something very special out of you. It requires no analysis, only presence. It is your form of expression. The form will vary but the message begs the simple formula:

Be present

Feel the pulse

Play

Know

There is no figuring-out process that opens the door to Wisdom. In fact, such an approach slows the journey, while giving the illusion of control and knowledge. Figuring something out is about pouring knowledge in. Finding Wisdom is about creating emptiness or quiet so that nothing can overwhelm what is already present, but potentially hidden from view.

Coach's Tip: If you are spending time "figuring out" what course of action serves your Highest Self, stop! Instead, get quiet, pose the question to which you want insight, connect with something you love, and wait—in silence, open to what possibilities come your way.

Many people will pray for help and then say they didn't get an answer. Is it that no guidance or path was suggested, or that the one praying expected the answer to come in a specific way so did not or could not recognize the help when it was offered? Listening *for* Wisdom means recognizing that there is a power beyond your own mind. It means that you may need to learn to listen *to* different kinds of messages in order to recognize the Wisdom. One tremendous source is your body.

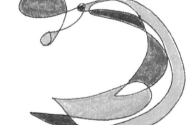

Listen to your body

When you are trying to discern wisdom from noise, one particularly helpful approach is to pay attention to whether your body is resisting your proposed direction or course of action. People register intuition in different places in their bodies. Three familiar places are the stomach, hands, and chest. Your body is wired to tell you the truth about whether what you are thinking supports your path and Highest Self or not.

At the most basic level, notice how your body responds when you make a declaration, such as, "I'm quitting my job tomorrow." Do your palms sweat? Does your stomach churn? Does your chest get tight or feel heavy? On the other hand, perhaps your chest opens and you feel light and free at the thought of quitting. Consider the possibility that your body may be signaling what choice produces dis-ease as opposed to ease in your life. How you respond comes later. What matters now is that you are attuned to the messages and not distracted by focusing on the "shoulds" in your head.

It is a simple approach. People have written extensively about how we register Wisdom in our bodies. Tools such as applied kinesiology[2] and visual journaling[3] are also used to help you attune to what your body is trying to signal you.

The principle is really quite simple. The heart knows your path. To the extent you are listening to and following its wisdom, your body moves with ease to support you. To the extent you tell yourself that something is true and then make choices that are inconsistent with that "truth," you produce stress and dis-ease in the body. For example, if you know that your voice is shut down in a relationship, whether at work or home, and you tell yourself to get over it and that it doesn't matter—and it does—your body will try to signal you that you are lying to yourself.

To the extent that you continue to bully your Self and deny the body's messages, you create resistance and dis-ease in your body. You know in your heart—and every cell of your body—what direction and choices support your Highest Self. Creative distractions of the mind are no more than noise. To the extent you feed those distractions, you direct your energy to work twice as hard denying what you know to be true. In time, the body won't put up with your games because it is a part of that wonderful conspiracy to support living into your highest potential. Lying to your Self is not a part of that plan. If you want the path of ease and joy, then you will need to return to the silence in which Wisdom appears, and remove yourself from the unconscious mind that wants to preserve the status quo relationships that may not be serving you.

In silence, the answers are revealed, even if they don't appear to be answers when you first start. Let go of expectations. Create a fertile space. Stay open to whatever appears. Continue to notice what gets your attention, name it, and move on. Test whether you are hearing the Inner Voice by remaining attuned to the messages and signals of your body in terms of relative ease or dis-ease. When words or signals come to you, you may find it helpful to write them in a journal, or find some other form of creativity where you express what is inside that wants expression. Without critical judgment, engage the child's sense of wonder at what will come out if you create the space for deep listening and creative expression.

EXERCISE TO BY-PASS THE MIND AND TUNE-IN TO WISDOM

I learned this exercise, which I found to be invaluable, in a workshop on intuition, led by Rosalie Deer Heart some years ago. It is called non-dominant journaling. It is a basic tool for allowing your rational mind to have a conversation with your Highest Self.

Your dominant hand is the one with which you write or throw a ball. Your non-dominant hand is the other one.

- Sit with a journal, or blank paper, prepared to have a conversation.

- With your dominant hand, write the question into which you seek insight.

Hint: This is not the place for simple "yes-no," or choices that are not particularly critical to your path and Best Self—like whether to buy the red or green car. Sample questions to get you started, might be something like the following:

- What Wisdom do you have for me about this job choice?
- I don't know what to do about moving or staying. Any ideas?
- How can I tell whether to stay in this relationship?

- Once you have written the question, place your pencil or pen in your non-dominant hand and if nothing is in your head to write, write the words "thank you" repeatedly until other words pop into your head.

Some people will receive whole messages, some will write twenty "thank you's" before a word pops in. Be very careful not to analyze what you write, or to look for coherence in what you write. Consider yourself a scribe, getting down what you are given. If the "answers" you have written are not clear to you, ask follow-up questions such as:

- I'm having trouble understanding. Can you be more explicit?
- Is there more you want me to know on this topic?
- Am I getting the message? Is there something else I need to understand?

If you practice this exercise regularly, you are likely to write whole paragraphs, tune-into your intuition more easily, access your Inner Voice on critical issues, and avoid the temptation to "figure out" decisions that need to come from the heart. Do not analyze or interpret the non-dominant messages immediately. Put them away for a while and you will be more able to receive the Wisdom when you are not as tied to a specific answer.

Personal reflections on in-dwelling

I find I'm laughing at myself a lot these days, thinking I'm uncovering some brilliant insight, only to find it was there all along in song lyrics or other forms just waiting for me to awaken to it.

The journey inward is a humbling experience. It teaches how disconnected we can become by working to fit in or succeed by others' standards. It exposes how we actually come to believe that we control our lives, rather than recognizing other forces at play. Our identities are developed and reinforced by an outward focus and sometimes a genuine intention to make a difference. If we are unconscious, we begin to accept the views of outsiders as more true than the wisdom of our own hearts, and we build all sorts of resistance into our paths—paths that could be natural and easy if we were awake and listening to our Inner Wisdom.

Looking back on the years of focus on my inward journey, three of those years with three dedicated consecutive days of silence a month to exploring inner depths, I am grateful for the Wisdom granted and the accompanying lighthearted perspective on life. We really are a funny lot and it's wonderfully freeing to laugh continuously at my own assumptions and near misses, rather than feel guilty, fearful, or worried about exactly how I will be seen or evaluated.

The beauty of a journey into silence is the gift of perpetual optimism. There is a confidence that comes from knowing that you will always be supported in your journey to Highest Self, if you choose it. There is a gentle nudge that assuming credit for success in human terms is more than self-inflation; it's off the mark. Our journey is guided and if we seek help, it's there. The commitment required is the willingness to develop faith in the inspired truth of Inner Wisdom.

Joy is there for the asking—in silence and reconnection with heart's desire. Time is an illusion. I delight in changes I made in my life for reasons I didn't recognize at the time. For example, I left a wonderful contemporary condominium on the ocean to purchase a 300 year old home with narrow stairs, six foot ceilings, floors so bowed they seemed to flow straight into the harbor, and a myriad of charming impracticalities. I thought at the time I needed a change and wanted a fireplace. It turns out that this house was instrumental in slowing me down and promoting a higher level of consciousness. With staircases as narrow and steep as they were and door jams barely over five feet, I literally had to slow down and pay attention to what I was doing at all times or I would hurt myself!

What is fascinating is that I bought the house, after looking at homes for a few weeks, in literally two hours. It was an intuitive knowing that that place was right, even if logically it seemed impractical. It served my purpose at the time and definitely supported my journey inward, the process of in-dwelling. Other benefits of in-dwelling included a recognition of and deeper connection with the things that delight and fill me.

> *My own connection to nature is very deep—perhaps deeper than I ever really recognized. I've always appreciated the sun or moonlight on the ocean, sounds of the tides, sunsets—but there's more. I'm content to sense the essence of the marsh or marvel at the blue heron or spider.*

Reflecting on where my journey inward began to really take form and where I am today, I am struck by how much has changed on the inside. I am not really sure how many people, with the exception of those who were aware of what I was doing and who had been closely watching, would notice the change on the outside. I still do similar work but the person I bring to my work is very different. My voice has changed and is still developing as I continue my own journey, and interact with and learn from others.

I have become acutely aware of the extent to which I have allowed my head to overrun my heart, to distract me from my own wisdom and my own work in the world. Slowing down and valuing what is inside are proving to be invaluable gifts. Much of what I want to share is how to stay true to your own journey. The world needs us to be centered at this time in our history. We have such wonderful potential and such incredible gifts that it makes no sense to me to squander them on worlds of our own imaginings, distractions, and worries that are not "true." There are wise women, men, and children walking around today who support the best in everyone. They remind us of the opportunity to stand for our individual and collective Best Selves.

To help you prepare for your own in-dwelling process, I offer below a few of my journal entries from later phases of my journey inward.

I find myself seeking space to be quiet, alone with Spirit, removed from the hustle and bustle of today's media. The space within is filled with Beauty and inspiring art, quiet reflection. It's not a space deprived of anything, rather a more discerning eye has guided what would be fulfilling in terms of hearing heart's desire and what is disruptive or distracting.

What fascinates me is how vague the journey can be at the beginning—a vague sense of destination with little or no direct guidance of choices to be made along the way. The route's markings are not recognizable at the beginning because, in a sense, this journey is developing a whole new way to Be with Self. It's a meeting conducted through a language which has been foreign to me. So I would not have recognized the signals along the way. I would have tried to fit them into my prior mental models of how things are and how they are meant to be.

Three days of quiet was extreme in terms of the pace and focus of my life two-and-one-half years ago. I realize how important it was that the calling came through a channel I trusted implicitly, a wise advisor. Other attempts to get my attention had not been successful in getting me to go inward to reconnect with the Wisdom of my heart and get out of my head.

I realize how critical breaking the unconscious pattern of my life firmly, yet gently, and thoroughly was. It is so easy when operating at a less than fully conscious level to merely incorporate newness into old frames and not really appreciate what I am choosing or how I am being. Three days meant no exceptions—and I was used to making exceptions for others who were not comfortable with my choices. These days allowed no business, no contact, other than greeting people on my walks, and no "other focus." In the early days, I couldn't see why it had to be so extreme, but now I do. I recognize what I perceive when interacting with others and, rather than listening to my head just gloss over or bury what someone who matters to me might not see, I consciously listen to the guidance of my intuition for how to respond.

The journey is a settling in, a familiarizing and then building intimacy in relationship with Self that sheds light on how disconnected I had become from my Self. I could be whoever others needed me to be but I would be limiting my Self from stepping up. This new space inside feels warm, inviting with a constant flame burning, fluid, cozy, and very intimate. From this Center I can lead a more conscious life and thereby manifest more directly heart's desire because I am more in touch with it. Accessing my truth is a faster process than words would allow. It seems to bypass my brain and flow directly from cellular knowing to my voice.

It's the simple beauty of what is that inspires, calms, brings me back to my Center. For someone able to think at a rapid pace and move among a confluence of clients and services, I am very content to be—and do nothing. Presence takes full focus.

In-dwelling is a gift you give your Self and those whose lives you touch. It begins with the deep desire to reconnect with the passion and truth of who you are at your essence. Here is a quick summary of the **In-Dwelling Process:**

1. Create the space to go inward

    a. Give yourself permission to create quiet space—and do it

    b. Detach from a focus on "doing"

   c. Experience and pay attention to feelings and reactions
   d. Get comfortable with and build nurturing structures

2. *Shine the light on unconscious patterns and behaviors*

   a. Notice and name distractions—and move on
   b. Watch when you push versus pull
   c. Meditate to expand consciousness

3. *Discern Inner Wisdom from noise*

   a. Listen attentively for Inner Wisdom
   b. Nurture creative self expression
   c. Listen to your body

The gift of in-dwelling will be a place of inner peace where you know your own voice. The Inner Voice that serves to guide your path will become more familiar to you and more present as you determine what choices and relationships deserve your energy and focus. You have been preparing the soil for new growth. Now it is time to look carefully at what is growing in your garden and what you are nurturing with your energy and focus.

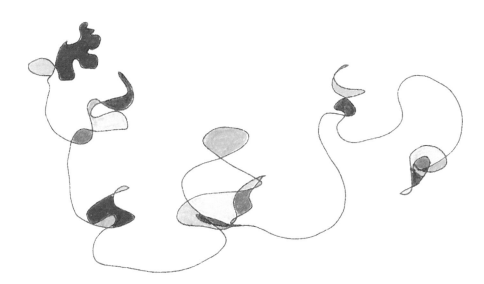

Before taking this step, let's pause to map your journey so far on the Universal Soul Grid.

Reflection Checklist

1. Know where you were

2. Know where you are

3. Know where you are headed

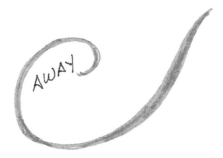

Where you were

When you picked up this book, you started back at Away with a vague sense of there being more to life than what you were experiencing. Whatever the prompts were in your life—changing personal relationships, life transition, less than fulfilling work situation, or just a sense of wanting more from your life—your wake-up call was beckoning.

The early prompts were signaling you that you needed to reconnect with the passion, desires, and Wisdom of your heart. The journey back to your Center called you to redirect your intensity and focus inward—to engage the process of in-dwelling. The process provided you the opportunity to reflect on who you have become and how you got there. You were provided the tools to create the space to go inward, to reconnect with your Highest Self. The process of shining light on the beliefs, thought patterns, "shoulds," and patterns of behavior that are no longer true for you allowed you to recognize the burdens and weights that you have been carrying for a long time. In reconnecting with your heart and its Wisdom, in listening to the intuitive messages that come your way, you have been invited to get reacquainted with your Highest Self.

Reconnecting with the freedom, lightness, joy, and exhilarating qualities that are inherent in your Highest Self gives you a touchstone for consciously knowing who you really are and what your life's path—purpose—is. As you spend more time creating space to hear the voice that is yours and knowing its truth, you continue to recognize different qualities of your Highest Self. You are beginning to understand how important it is to maintain that space for connection with your Highest Self, if you want to step into your potential and lead from your strengths. You are also more aware of the importance—in the moment—of paying attention to which people and situations nurture and help you give voice to that Highest Self, and which ones don't.

You are now in a place to more consciously choose to continue to deepen your relationship at Home with your Highest Self, feeling the peace and joy that is there for you. As you nurture that relationship over time, you will find yourself wanting to make that Highest Self a central part of your daily life. What is happening at this point in terms of where you are on the Soul Grid is that you have been inviting the process of in-dwelling to reconnect you with your Highest Self at the upper spiral of Home. Where we will focus next is on increasing your ability to bring your Highest Self into your everyday activities in a very conscious way. The movement will be outward from the upper spiral of Home towards the outward world of Away.

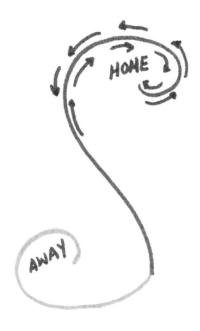

Where you are headed*
(*with any luck this is also where you want to be!)

The next process is the opposite of in-dwelling. You are now looking to integrate your Highest Self with external activities of daily life. Now that you are more consciously aware of the impact of choosing from your heart over your head, it is time to design your life to help you do this in every relationship you engage. You are ready to practice living consciously—by design.

Conscious living means that you are moving from the top spiral of the Soul Grid to the lower spiral of Away through a series of conscious steps and choices demanding your full and complete presence in each moment of your life.

By design means that you are consciously clarifying who you choose to be and how you express your Self in the world—developing and following a basic life architecture or a garden master plan with clear design principles (core values) and lots of room for details to change and emerge.

Conscious living means no opportunities for mindlessly going through the day. No matter what you are doing—brushing your teeth, laundry, washing the car, balancing your checkbook, conducting a business meeting, or whatever—you are paying attention to how you are *being* at that moment. You are watching for when your energy goes up and when you feel drained. You immediately recognize when your head introduces thoughts and you step back to evaluate whether or not to entertain them, rather than blindly following their seductive distraction from the experience of the moment. Your heart leads. Your head follows. In being present, you are walking the path of consciously making choices in your life that support bringing your Highest Self to all you are and to all you do. You are learning to be in today's hectic world without losing your Center. You are learning to become a beacon in the crowd, rather than muffling your voice and light to fit in. By being true to your Highest Self, you light the way for others to see their potential.

While Away, you continuously connect with your intuition and vigilantly guard against unconscious decisions to accumulate ego-identity relationships that tempt you with earthly measures of power, status, and validation. You develop the ability to express your authentic Self in a way that attracts to you relationships and opportunities that support your life's purpose and passions. As you go, you check back with Home and say good-bye to relationships that no longer serve you. And you do all of this from your heart—which means that whatever the qualities of your voice, they are rooted in truth and Inner Wisdom.

On this path, there is a potential stumbling block. Be forewarned. Just because you engage your journey and build your confidence to stay true to your passions, principles, and purpose does not mean that everyone who is or has been a part of your life is delighted with your choices. Those who do not want you to change will become distractions on your path if you let them. Note that there is no judgment here. They are not bad people doing bad things by judging you harshly, expressing their disapproval, or denying you support. Their behavior is about them—their fears and attachments. It is not about you.

Step back—with no judgment, meaning, or interpretation—and ask whether what these people say rings true in your heart. If so, consider the wisdom they offer. If not, stay the course and walk your path, always leaving room for others to gracefully reenter your life when it serves both of you again. Remember that if you stop on your path to take care of or rescue others so that they do not have to take care of themselves, you slow their journey, as well as your own. A simple question to ask your Self is whether the way you are responding is from your heart. If you respond from guilt, obligation, or "should," you have lost the connection with your heart. Be grateful to those who test your resolve because they create the opportunity for you to stay present, vigilant, committed to your path, and conscious of all your choices to say, "Yes."

You have been traveling inward in ways you probably haven't done for a long time, experiencing the magnificent garden that is your Highest Self. Now that you have cleared the path to step into the highest potential of your passions and Self, it is time to leave the inner sanctum and grow this magnificent garden in every aspect of your daily life. As you return to the everyday concerns of Away, you bring the clarity and beauty of your Best Self—your rich and lush garden, your Home—into each situation and relationship that you encounter.

One more thing. As you journey back into the world of expectations and social convention, pay attention to every request for your time, attention, and energy. Make conscious choices about what nurtures your garden and feeds the very Best in you. The goal is to return an even more **whole you** to everyday decisions and relationships, prepared to be the person you choose and to walk your true path every day. Ready? Check your supplies. Do you have what you need?

Coach's Tip: Leave the Critic behind. Bring the Child.

As you design the life you choose to live and the person you choose to be in every moment, you will need to carry with you the open-eyed wonder of a child. The child—before adults train her or him otherwise—sees the beauty in what is, because the child is not distracted by the human world of "shoulds". The wonder and awe of life are not lost on a child. It is the child's perspective that will ground you, that will remind you to remain connected with your heart.

By contrast, the critic in each of us is trained to see and find gaps. No matter how wonderful something is, the critic proves her or his worth by identifying something amiss or missing. For those of you who have chosen professions that train you to look for gaps—law, accounting, and audit, for example—you will need to be extra vigilant to recognize the critic's voice drowning the Wisdom of the child.

For those of you still hooked on an ego-identity of being right, you need more in-dwelling to look more closely at why you think your relationship with correctness serves your Highest Self. For the rest, send your resident critic—who lives rent-free in your head—on vacation. Carry your child with you—she's a lifeline to your heart.

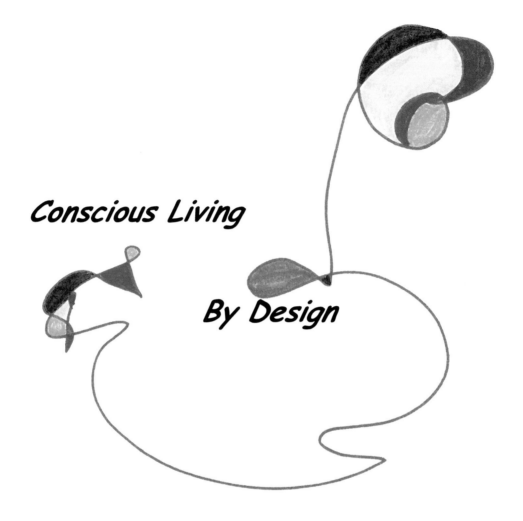

Conscious Living

By Design

Away we go—conscious, alive, and awake to all that life offers! This next phase of the journey is about how to **be _in_ the world without being _of_ it.** It's about connecting with your own light and Grace in such a way that you light up from within and don't look for others to provide light for you. You do not look for happiness from a partner in a relationship because you know that you carry your own happiness within you. Your happiness is what you bring to a relationship, not what you expect the relationship to provide you. The joy and inner peace that you experience when you carry all that is Home inside you allows you to be with others who are suffering through difficult challenges without internalizing the pain yourself. You respond with compassion, not sympathy. Your boundaries are so clear that you can offer love and appreciation without feeling others' pain, as if it were your own. You can travel in dark places with shady characters and not lose your way because who you are does not change. When you live this path consistently, you are free, light, and able to dance with the rhythm of Life itself, open to whatever comes your way.

What does it take to design your life to support conscious and enlightened living? Four basic steps:

Design your garden for growth
Step into your Grace
Speak from your heart
Lead from Wisdom

Let's begin with the first step:

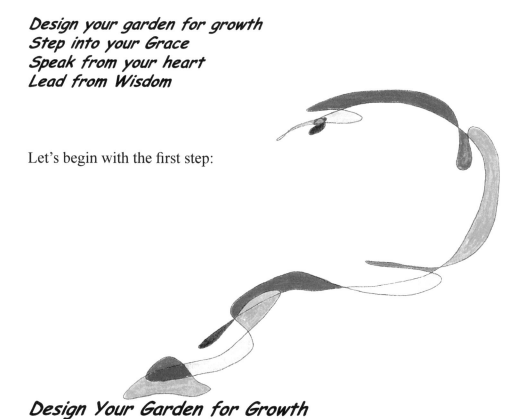

Design Your Garden for Growth

The in-dwelling process supports your getting quiet and discerning the truth in your heart. If you can achieve stillness in moments of every day, you can begin to hear the Wisdom of your heart more clearly above the din of outside demands in your everyday world. The initial connection with your Highest Self gives you a sense of the potential magnificence of your own garden. To foster that magnificence, you will need to look more carefully at what is growing in your current life and what wants growth—your heart's desires. A great place to develop the aerial view of what you are currently growing in your garden is to look at all the ***relationships*** that make up your life today and assess which ones energize you, fill your heart, and move you towards your Highest Self, and which ones drain more energy than they give back. In essence, you are developing a master plan for your garden by looking at what your soil easily and joyfully supports, as opposed to what drains it of its nutrients and beauty.

Any relationship—whether with another individual, group, tribe, country, idea, belief system, or work— is a wonderful mirror through which you see your Self. Since none of us exists in isolation, who you become in every relationship reveals how much you lead your life from your head versus your heart. To the extent you know your Best Self and have a clear intention about how you want to express that Self, you are prepared to make healthy choices that support your potential. Your garden flourishes! To the extent you are not very clear, you are destined to create entanglements and dependencies that satisfy external expectations and ego-identity. The life of joy—the magnificent and lush garden that is yours— requires that you look carefully at where you are growing weeds and entanglements that are choking the life out of your garden.

We are coming into a time in history where we cannot afford to expend any energy in relationships that are not healthy. The bombardment of media messages, pressure to do everything faster, and increased focus on doing more with fewer resources are testing our ability to remember who we are at our Center and what we really believe. If you jump into unconscious partnerships and other relationships without asking what you want from them and at what cost, you are likely to use your valuable energy maintaining relationships that drain your life force. Relationships that support Best Self are worth energy. Those that don't support Best Self need to go away. This doesn't necessarily mean that the people, situation, or work has to go away. It means that how you relate to it needs to change.

Coach's Tip: Every relationship represents a choice.

How many of yours are conscious choices?

> *Once created, the relationship (with Highest Self) requires constant attention and nurturing, as does any relationship you want to sustain. The next step in the process is to integrate that relationship in your external relationships in a way that it guides you in making decisions from your Center, grounded in the Wisdom that you know to be true. It is a journey of faith. And that faith will be tested.*

When you have touched your Center, you consciously know the wholeness of life and the peace that fills and surrounds your Highest Self. You recognize your truth and Wisdom and will find you want to hold onto it. You know how precious it is. Staying in touch with the sense of magic and oneness that is your Highest Self often registers as an overwhelming desire to act with integrity, to preserve the integrity that is you in all of your choices. It begins to drive a new awareness about relationships in your life—at every level—as you weigh decisions about how to invest your energy and focus in order to nurture your passions and Highest Self, rather bury them again.

Living into your Highest Self means living from your strengths and gifts in all parts of your life. If you recognize that there are contexts where your Best Self doesn't fit or thrive, the question is not how to hide those qualities. The question is why you are selecting to focus any energy in those contexts or relationships.

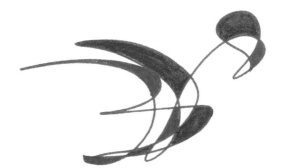

See the relationship for what it is

In beginning a new or redesigning a current relationship, your clarity about what you are willing to invest and what you want back from any given relationship affects whether and how you choose to be in the relationship. If you are intentional about who you chose to be in the relationship—light hearted, playful, joyful, intense, competent, or any other qualities—then you can more clearly assess whether being in a particular relationship in the way that relationship works is fulfilling your desires or falling short.

Such clarity makes it easier to tell the truth about what you want from the relationship and also to articulate boundaries about what you will give and what you require in order to sustain the relationship. If you are not clear about who you choose to be in life and how you want to express your truth, you can choose to cut your heart off from expressing your truth and allow the voices in your head to convince you that you are asking for too much, being unreasonable, or ungrateful. You may shut down the truth, focus instead on what you want to believe about the situation, and foster a relationship that robs you of your connection with your Highest Self. The choice is about consciousness and the decision to determine which relationships truly nurture your Best Self. The alternative is to avoid facing what drains you and hope that "things will change" on their own. Any relationship unconsciously maintained takes a tremendous amount of energy and life force. Are you ready to free your Self from entanglements that no longer serve you?

Many people believe it is too much work and too scary to look squarely at relationships they know are not fulfilling to them. Many are afraid that if they see a relationship for what it is, they will have to deal with it. But for those who are clear about who they want to be, what they want to stand for, or what they want to create in their lives, seeing and dealing with relationships that don't align with Best Self is imperative. Denial is simply unproductive and costly when you have developed the capacity and desire for the truth that serves a life of joy and ease.

> *Detachment from what others think will affect my relationships—some to the point of good-bye. Others may feel they no longer know me. What is clear needs to be within me and to serve as my compass for decisions.*

You become more open to the truth of what is when you are able step back from how you want things to look, sound, feel, and be and look squarely at what is. When you are able to step back and get some perspective on a relationship, your mind's judgments are slowed down to hear the body's reactions. Do you tense up at the mention of a boss' voicemail or e-mail? Your body may signal a level of fear and power that you give your boss that is worth testing against what you know in your heart. Are you telling yourself that you are only good enough when you please him or her? Are you clear about what you agree to give in the relationship and what you get back? Detaching from how you think you should react is what will allow you to hear the truth in your heart—to access your own intuition. Your Inner Voice becomes loud enough for you to recognize its message about any relationship you may be involved in or considering entering.

In the work world today, we are more often rewarded for quick thinking and mental acuity than for intuition and heart wisdom. While your heart and body don't lie, your head might in order to preserve the status quo. If you live a good part of your life in your head and your identity is related to having a particular position, power base, or level of intelligence as judged by others, there is a good possibility that you override your intuition unconsciously to avoid having to change your relationship with anything that feeds your identity.

For example, imagine that you tell your Self that a work situation really isn't all that bad and that you can stay until you retire by laying low and collecting your paycheck. But when you state this belief, your chest feels like a weight is pressing on it, or your stomach churns, and your throat tightens. Consider that your body is trying desperately to get you to be honest with your Self. Deep down you know that you will not be able to disengage and just collect a paycheck. The decision to do so is going to cost you in many ways, not the least being your physical and mental health. Using your body in this way to test whether the decision about a current relationship is in support of your Highest Self is something anyone who wants the truth can do.

EXERCISE TO CHECK UNEASINESS

This exercise can be applied in almost any context to immediately tune into your body signals. The next time you feel uneasy but are not sure of the exact source of the unease:

- Pause for a minute.

- Pay attention to what you have just told yourself—or another person.

- Repeat that message and notice any body signals.

- Where are you registering a response—uneasiness—in your body?

- Did you become defensive, compassionate, or indignant when you acted the way that brought on this body reaction?

- How do these qualities compare with who you are when you are your Highest Self?

Now step back again and notice what message in your head supported the behavior your body does not support.

- What were you thinking at the time your body registered the response?

- What relationship do you have with the message or its source?

- Why do you give it such power? What are you afraid will happen if you don't?

Once you have answered these questions, remember not to judge yourself. You don't need to "do" anything; just notice what is happening when it happens. Notice what relationship fosters the dis-ease in your body.

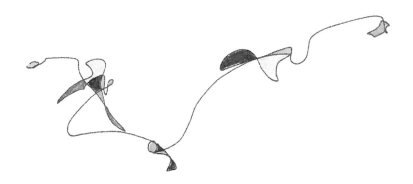

Some relationships may need to go. The people, work, or aspects of the situation in which you find your Self may stay, but how you relate to them will change. If those with whom you are in relationship are unwilling to support the changes you need to make, then you may need to be prepared to leave the relationship behind. But remember, no one is forcing you to make the change. You choose how you respond to every relationship in your life. If you do not follow your Inner Wisdom, more and more energy will be required to hold onto unhealthy relationships, leaving you unavailable for healthy ones.

In Western society, we typically don't pay attention to who we are becoming and what is really going on in our lives until we are forced to do so. Some people are so skilled at not seeing that it takes either loss of a major relationship—job loss, divorce, death—or a personal illness to get their attention. We have become so preoccupied with linear goals and expectations that once we achieve them, we forget that everything grows and changes. We spend incredible amounts of energy trying to preserve the relationships as they once were or as we have wanted them to be. Even relationships that are healthy at one point become unhealthy if the members do not acknowledge how they are changing and what that means for the relationship.

A relationship grows organically as each individual grows and changes. If you do not see yourself as at least half of the equation and evaluate what you want from and choose to contribute to the relationship as well as what is returned to you, the likelihood that you become either too controlling or too passive is high. Your ability to grow into your Best Self diminishes. One sure indicator of shifting needs in a relationship is the recognition that what was once a perfectly appealing and desirable trait of the other party in the relationship has become a burden or thing of lesser value.

For example, I once owned a beautiful old home with harbor views from every floor and terraced gardens in the backyard. For several years, that wonderful haven served to help me to slow down and live into different aspects of my life. Then I reached a stage in my life where keeping up an old home and gardening became chores. The beautiful gardens that were once a selling point in the relationship I had with my home became more of a cost when I found myself spending more time maintaining than enjoying them. Others told me I was crazy to sell this charming home, but I knew it was time. What my heart told me to do did not fit with the recommendations of others who could only see the charm of my home, and not how it fit within my life's changing priorities. What I found to be true applies to all of us. The message within needs to be absolutely clear or the voices of convention will prevail. And when they do, you will spend energy in ways that do not serve you—but which look good to others.

The same thing happens at work. You may join an organization for one reason and stay because it seems to be the path of least resistance. Yet, without conscious attention to what is coming back to you, it becomes easier to convince your Self that staying is less costly than leaving. Are you overlooking the cost to inner peace and Highest Self? Are you trying to convince yourself that you have to stay or that you have no choice? Look carefully at all the energy you are investing in not seeing the relationship as it is.

BODY PULSE EXERCISE

This exercise is a follow-up to discerning uneasiness in your body. The focus here is on what you are investing and what you are getting back from every relationship in which you engage. As you ponder the following questions, pay attention to your body's reaction to your responses.

- What are you getting back for the emotional energy that you invest, dreams you share, and time you spend?

- Are you becoming more of the person you like or drifting away from your Best Self?

Repeat this exercise as often as you like until you can clearly identify what relationships you are spending time watering, caring for, and feeding that do not belong in a garden that supports your highest potential.

In reflecting on how you spend your energy, you may find that you spend an incredible amount of that energy on keeping a relationship going with someone who neither understands nor values the (zany and outrageous?) person you are at your core. To maintain the relationship, you shut your Self down to fit the way this other person wants you to be. You further recognize that you have been telling your Self that it is unreasonable to expect him to understand or appreciate this side of you. You tell your Self that he is good for you even as you feel your stomach knot and a lump form in your throat when you begin to say what is in your heart. Naming what you see and experience in the pit of your stomach and in your throat gives voice to your truth. You can then decide what to do about what you see. It may be time to weed the garden.

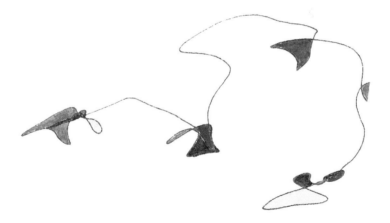

Weed and prune the garden

To be your Best Self in all that you are and all that you do requires constant focus and care, just as the garden does, in order to not become overrun by one specific plant or weed. The weeds and unwanted other elements in the garden are relationships, beliefs, thought patterns, and ways of being and doing that choke the growth out of the garden. They rob it of its ability to flourish. Without constant clarity about what the garden is to be, you will find it easily overrun by plants that creep into parts of the garden where they don't belong.

Every relationship—whether with work, thoughts, beliefs, or people—is a seed with the potential to grow. It is safe to say that the seed does not sprout immediately. It takes time, and during the season of developing roots, nothing is visible above the surface. The roots go down before the flower comes up. Each relationship develops roots. Some relationships in our lives take up a lot of room in our garden. Maybe they are emotionally draining or demanding in terms of what it takes to support their growth. Maybe they are just big and demand lots of space. The point here is that the garden is designed by the gardener—you! And if you don't like what is growing, it is up to you to change it.

One of the challenges is that your garden has been around for a long time and many of the plants and weeds have very deep roots—usually undiscovered until you attempt to remove or transplant them. Once you have decided what kind of garden you will support, what kind of person you choose to be in all that you do, it is time to step back and really look carefully at what is growing, what is thriving, and what is being choked out by other relationships. With your intention clear, detach, and name the quality and characteristics of those relationships.

RELATIONSHIP INVENTORY EXERCISE

Sometimes it helps to have a graphic depiction of what is going on. The following exercise gives you a picture of how you currently invest your energy in relationships.

1. Draw a circle on a sheet of paper.
2. Separately from that circle, make four headings on a sheet of paper—Home, Work, Others, and Self.
3. Identify what proportion of your energy and time goes into each of these four areas in the waking hours of each week.
4. Map all four of them relative to each other on the circle by dividing up the pie of energy you have available for relationships into where you invest that energy today.

With the pie chart in front of you, consider the following questions:

- How is the pie divided?

- Are you spending time and energy in relationships that give back to you at least as much as what you put into them?

- If the answer is "no," beware of any excuses you tell your Self for why not!

- What proportion of the pie today supports your relationship with Self? Is it enough to nurture your soul and propel the very best in you forward? Is it enough to keep you connected with Wisdom, joy, and ease?

- Where are you focusing too much attention?

- Where do you need more?

This exercise provides you with a quick "aerial view" of your garden. How does it look? Is it designed to support all that is best and highest in you? Consider where pruning and weeding would help.

If you are not absolutely clear about the person you are choosing to be and are unwilling to look at where you are investing your emotional energy, you are not ready to let go of what is limiting you and making you less than fulfilled in your life. If you *are* ready, then the process is one of naming what you see and determining if and where a given relationship fits in your life—effectively weeding the garden in service of Highest Self and your life's work.

When you can name beliefs that you have held for as long as you remember and admit that they no longer serve you, ask yourself whether you are ready to pull them up by their roots. If not, what do you need to do to appreciate how they have gotten you this far, and release them? The same is true for any kind of loyalty that no longer serves the person you choose to be. Be completely and compassionately honest with your Self. The core question to ask your Self is whether it matters more to you that you are true to your Best Self or that others are happy with and validate you. *Are you designing your garden to support your passions or your distractions?*

These are not easy questions and not questions to be asked only once. In this weeding process, you will ask your Self these questions about all of your relationships many times. What makes weeding the garden more doable is that it is driven by clarity, love, and the passion you have to nurture your Best Self. Serving that Best Self becomes clearer and easier the more you courageously stand for the person you want to be, rather than giving your power to other people or ways of thinking that replace your light with fear and doubt.

Look closely—and fearlessly.

Nurture what serves you.

Weed out what doesn't.

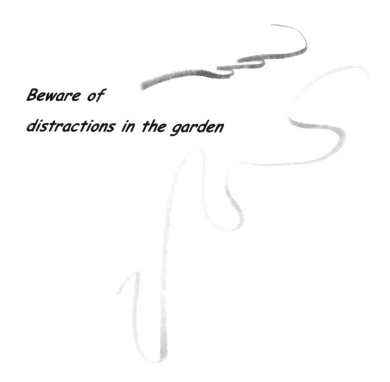

Beware of

distractions in the garden

There are distractions that may appear as you attempt to weed the garden. Remember that the mind has not given up trying to maintain the status quo. In its quest to keep you in line, it will offer roles—complete with scripts—that you may choose to play out, rather than telling your Self the truth about what you are and are not getting back from your relationships with people, ideas, beliefs, and organizations. Here are three of the more common ones.

The victim

In this role, you cast your Self as being robbed of your power by things and people's actions beyond your control. Acting the role involves some internal dialogue to convince your Self that the way you believe the world should work, and the way you get to be in it are reasonable and just. Any reality that does not support your beliefs is somehow flawed. It is someone else's fault that you are not happy or not your Best Self.

In the victim role, you practice a kind of blindness and lying to your Self that absolves you of any accountability for your choices, sometimes to the point where you convince your Self that you do not actually have any choice. When confronted, the most practiced victims will usually respond with some form of denial, as in, "That's not a real choice. I didn't have any choice." If the internal dialogue continues long enough, you convince your Self that you have no choice but to stay in work that is not meaningful or fulfilling, relationships that stifle creativity and self-expression, and a life that brings anything but joy. You abandon the choice to approach your relationships with work, with the world, and with other people as your own best advocate, as you become an unconscious sleepwalker in your relationships.

The victim is rewarded with sympathy and protection in our society, precisely because behaving as a victim allows others to hide from themselves. It is much easier to be supportive of someone you perceive as an underdog than to take a stand for reminding that individual that she or he has a choice in creating a satisfying life. When you fail to raise others up and remind them of their greatness, you collude in maintaining a victim role for yourself and them. You end up supporting relationships centered on pain and struggle, spending energy in conversations about all that is wrong in this world and what is not fair. Your relationship to what exists in the world is one of resistance. You retreat to the theatre in your head and foster a negative spiral of shoulds that allow you to be the victim.

When you take a stand for your own and others' greatness, you give others the opportunity to confront their own realities more clearly. If they admonish you for being unsympathetic, try pausing before you respond. You are at a choice point of either feeding a relationship that plays to your fears and ego, or shifting to one that nurtures your joy. Will you be a victim to your head's distractions and foster relationships that are not healthy and vibrant? When you play the victim role, you fail to recognize the game of collusion to avoid your own light and, therefore, accountability for your choices and lot in life.

The martyr

Another way not to see your Self as a co-creator of any relationship in which you enter is to take the part of the martyr. The martyr has transferred the value of Self to external sources, such as family, friends, colleagues, neighbors, or performance management systems, for approval. The martyr will often do what is expected in relationships but doesn't calculate the cost of his or her behavior to Self or the relationship. The martyr seeks and usually demands recognition for putting up with behavior or situations that she or he finds undesirable, rather than leaving or renegotiating the relationships.

The whole concept of leaving the relationship is foreign to the martyr. The martyr values the dependency on him or her in order to be able to complain about or gather kudos for putting up with such circumstances. Although the martyr would likely deny making such a choice, the martyr unwittingly ensures his or her own misery by choosing to be in relationships that are less than desirable, often to gain approval or attention. Some martyrs show up in the workplace as people who stay up all night to work on a big project, send e-mails at all hours, and then seek attention for those behaviors from colleagues. The alternative would be conscious choice and ownership for what one wants in and from the relationship—and then taking a stand for personal boundaries and expectations.

The bully or abuser

While the two previous forms of Best Self denial are roles that often garner empathy or sympathy from others because they play a less than active role in the relationship, the bully or abuser works a little differently. Still a form of denying Self in the relationship, the bully takes a more aggressive role, often declaring his or her judgments about a situation or decision to be supreme or preferred.

The bully wears a mask of being certain about the right way, the way things should be done, or ways a person should behave. The individual sets about making sure she or he sets the agenda and controls what others can and cannot do. The bully tends to hide fears from others through more aggressive behavior. Many who feel like imposters in all or parts of their life assume this role unwittingly in a wide variety of settings.

Rather than share the beauty of emotional vulnerability and self-discovery with others in the relationship, the bully or abuser feels the need to protect himself or herself from being discovered to be less than desired or not good enough. The role keeps people at a distance and gives the illusion of being in control and somehow better than others. The behaviors used to create and maintain this mask also make it difficult for others to express love and compassion towards the bully, who insulates himself or herself from the possibility that others might see through the disguise. All of this is to say that the hard edge others experience from the bully/abuser is a mask created out of fear that others might get too close or alternatively never choose to be close enough. For the bully, the relationship with Highest Self is absent, with no connection to what is possible when living from the heart.

In a society that is less than fully present, we do not calculate the cost of these roles on our lives. The roles of victim, martyr, bully, or any other role we might assume that diminishes being our Best Selves all the time, appear to be easier because we are only looking at immediate comfort in the situation. When we engage the ego and act out these roles, we are acting out a learned script, not conscious of who we are at our Center.

The antidote to unconscious and energy-consuming relationships is to choose your relationships with clarity of intention. At the point where you are able to shine the light on your adopted roles and patterns of behavior, you can more easily declare whether the relationship you are in is one that is distracting you from your life's path or supporting your Highest Self. If you want to live *your* life, it is critical that you know and be true to your Best Self by choosing to engage only in relationships that bring out that Best Self. By being more conscious of the choices you make and why you make them, you build your willingness to see the truth of your current situation. That willingness makes it easier to recognize what needs to be removed or cut back in your garden.

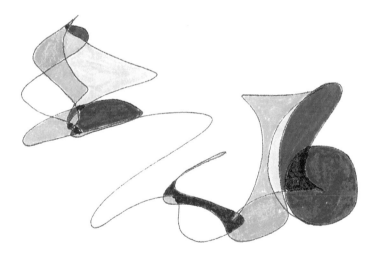

Prepare for goodbyes

Weed killers may well represent the kinds of structures that need to be designed into my life to prevent the ground from even being receptive to weed energies. Return the entanglements and unhealthy relationships to their rightful owners.

The letting go process, which is the moving-on stage, involves two elements: saying goodbye to relationships that need to go and tilling the soil to attract what you want. There is no magic formula for letting go, but one clear step is to notice what distractions your mind uses to perpetuate unhealthy or painful relationships. Choosing guilt over your Best Self is an example of a mind distraction that supports such relationships. Take a good look at the role guilt plays in your life. What are you afraid you would lose if you stopped feeling guilty? Who are you afraid of becoming if you step into your potential? Until you can answer these questions, you are not ready to reclaim your own power. Letting go is tremendously freeing if your focus is on what you want to create and not on how others might react.

It is a matter of your knowing who you want to be and what you are willing to both give and receive in the relationship. The relationship that needs to end is more often resolved by shifting your way of being with the person, work, or belief than by leaving the other party. Consider carefully the relationship's place in your life and how it contributes to your being your Best Self. Even a good thing can become unhealthy.

> *...also important to prune back overgrowth that is crowding out other plants from the light. Even the most beautiful need to be trimmed back for the sake of the whole garden...There are going to be some goodbyes in this process—weights I don't need and can't carry to be on (my) purpose.*

It is a time to be both firm and patient with your Self. Letting go may be difficult. Familiarity is much easier to deal with than the unknown if you are not fully awake to the choices you have been making and to the overall quality of your life. Staying in relationships that no longer support your Best Self and the contribution you want to make in the world is costly—on every level.

Remember that the energy you spend on any relationship in your life—on anything you are supporting or maintaining—is not available to you to grow something new. Continue to take an honest inventory of the relationships in your life that take your energy away rather than fill you up. You can do it by using the Energy Tracking Exercise at the end of the day to reflect on what activities, conversations, or people made you smile, brought you light, or energized you. Then reflect on what dragged you down, frustrated you, or emotionally engaged you in ways that did not bring out the best in you. Make a few notes in a journal and by the end of a week you will have a pretty good idea of what you need to do to support a flourishing garden.

> *There is something wonderfully freeing and beautifully creative in destroying the old that is not needed. I could feel the energy...If I care about the comfort of those I help in a way that causes me to hold back, I don't help them move forward.*

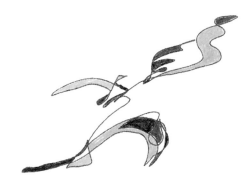

Design for new relationships

So what does it take to design for new relationships? If you choose to live a life where you approach everything with a light heart and humor, step back to observe every situation, belief, thought pattern, personal and professional relationship in terms of lightheartedness and humor. Ask your Self who you become when you are in these relationships. Does the path of least resistance lead to humor, or do you more often find your Self in situations where you are serious or intense? If your Best Self is loving and nurturing, do you find yourself in relationships where you both give and receive love? Do you get to nurture others and be nurtured in return? Or do you find you are making excuses for why others cannot or do not return the love and nurturing ways you so value?

If, for instance, you are most likely to be lighthearted and fun with people who are less serious themselves, create an opportunity to spend time with them and see how it goes. Then, with a designer's eye, notice what characteristics of that relationship you can extrapolate and reinsert into a different relationship to see whether you can be more of who you want to be in a different context. Continue the process. You are essentially trying on new skin. The pattern will reinforce itself naturally with practice and focus.

The more you laugh and approach situations more lightly, for example, the more you will find others responding to your lightness. You will find yourself naturally choosing situations and people who respond easily to your Best Self. As this continues, you will eventually find that you have less and less time and energy for those relationships that do not feed your Best Self. You may also find that your creativity increases in finding ways to evoke others' Best Selves just by being more true to the best in you. It becomes rather fun!

Recognize that you will attract opportunities to practice the new you with people who are used to your responding or behaving in ways that you may no longer choose. The first step is conscious awareness of who you are with those people or in those situations. Over time, if you choose to remain in the relationships, you will need to reframe the relationships and change how you behave with the same people. For now, notice what you experience, celebrate the small successes, and feel the growth inside.

Just noticing that you make a choice differently today than you might have made it yesterday is a beginning when designing new relationships. You have been shining light on unconscious thought patterns so that you can keep those that work for you and recognize those that don't. Be patient. Just because you recognize a thought pattern that isn't working doesn't mean you can release it immediately. It took a while to learn it and it will take a while to unlearn it. Stop judging and stay vigilant if you want to accelerate your ability to shift your choices in the moment to be more aligned with the person you know you want to be all the time.

> *I need to be very aware of my intentions and where I put my energy. Without careful discernment and attention, I could be "watering the weeds" (feeding the complainers, people who don't want to grow and change) and crowd out a potentially gorgeous garden.*

The exciting thing is that success builds on success. You become a magnet for the kinds of opportunities, ways of thinking, and relationships that serve your Best Self, which in turn helps you help others do the same thing. Sometimes, a Wisdom greater than your own helps you with circumstances that you may not recognize as favorable at the time. Relationships that fall away, jobs that disintegrate, or opportunities that you expect to materialize that don't are all examples. They may be clearing the way for new growth. Stay clear in your intention to cultivate a magnificent garden. Look carefully at what is going away. Before you invest any extra energy in trying to hold onto a relationship that you are afraid to lose, tune into your heart. If you can quiet your head long enough and trust the process, you may discover that what is happening is helping you on your journey—even if you don't like it at the time! Eventually, you can begin to laugh at your demands that something happen exactly as you picture it in the time frame you expect. It's uncanny how the timing of what truly benefits our path is exactly what we need—even if we do not recognize it as such!

I was laid off from work on two different occasions from different companies. In each case I faced financial challenges, and the prospect of finding a new job in very tight job markets with less than conventionally desirable skills or resume. In the first case, I was in a new geography with an expensive apartment and almost no savings. The economy was in recession and companies were not hiring. Because the company I was with went out of business, my network disappeared, and I had no idea whom to ask for help. A former client, who had been through layoffs, guided me through the process. In the end, another client found me a job at a better salary than I had been making and the whole picture changed in less than two months.

In the second case, I had been in senior management in different roles. In time, it became increasingly apparent that my strengths did not match the culture or goals of the organization. I wish I could tell you that I had the courage to follow my heart and leave, but I didn't. With little remaining clarity or confidence, I needed help out the door! Within weeks, I landed a role in an organization that was a wonderful match, used my experience, and gave me a chance to refine my skills and rebuild my confidence.

In both cases, I ended up better off for having left the "secure" position. The jobs that I worked so hard to maintain were actually eroding my Best Self, but I could not—or would not—see it at the time. I was trapped in conventional belief systems operating below my level of awareness, afraid to trust my heart. It doesn't need to be this way for you. Too many people today leave jobs and careers feeling deflated and questioning their strengths. Conscious choices to support Highest Self change that.

Who you become when you make choices that give you energy is someone more naturally able to move easily with what comes your way. Your energy is not tied up in trying to be what others expect or want you to be. You feel free to be your Self. Others experience your freedom as you begin to attract to you people who respond well to the Highest Self that you are now expressing. You more easily release old ways of thinking and behaving that don't support you, and begin to see relationships and opportunities through new eyes.

Coach's Tip: When you are true to who you are at your core, you attract people to your genuine Self—not who you think they want you to be. You are designed to flourish.

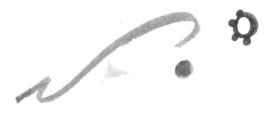

LILA'S RELATIONSHIP STORY

Lila worked in a corporate environment for a very long time. A wildly creative and playful person, she would constantly find ways to lighten the business environment, while demonstrating tremendous skill in getting her work accomplished. She insulated those she managed from less than talented leaders and effectively worked the system to get her department's work accomplished.

In time, however, the amount of energy and effort she expended to create a receptive environment increased to the point of negatively impacting her health. As her physical health deteriorated, her ability to sustain an environment that could hold her staff up began to wane and it became clear to her that she needed to leave the corporate position or lose her health. The relationship with work was costing far more than it was returning to Lila. She planned her exit and then left. She began carefully assessing all of the relationships in her life and choosing which ones to engage and how. The first relationships that she recognized as supporting her Highest Self were with nature, art, and her young children.

As she created a magical environment in her home with her young children, she found that she also began to attract corporate types who did not know how to play. They wanted to learn how to relax and be more creative. She started magnetizing relationships that reinforced her own shift to be more of who she truly is at her core without trespassing on the readiness of others to change.

One clear piece of wisdom that she followed was to create relationships in which she could express socially bold positions and behaviors usually relegated to children—not childish but childlike in their wonder, awe, and lightness—in subtle ways that intrigued and enticed adults. In this way, she inspired others to see the truth of what delights them.

In striking out in this direction she found that the process was not always easy. Lila encountered loneliness when she focused on finding others who both appreciated her Best Self and wanted to bring themselves to the relationship as full participants. The people who had been a part of her life, outside of her immediate family, did not really fit the new criteria. The loneliness caused her to examine the city in which she lived and her relationship to it. She learned to look closely at what she wanted in her life.

Today she is consciously re-establishing her tribe by identifying the kinds of people who support her authenticity and freedom to be her Self. She has noticed that she is no longer attracting those who want to be rescued. Her selection of friends and people with whom she engages continues to grow, at the same time as it narrows and screens out social climbers who are not aligned with the kinds of relationships worthy of her energy and health. Her connection with nature and artistic expression remain priorities, as she integrates those activities with family and friends. Integration of her Highest Self in her relationships and activities is critical.

It is important to note that engaging in nature walks and artistic endeavors doesn't mean that she is separating her Self from others. Quite the opposite! She is finding that knowing who she is at her core is making it easier to do the things she loves to do with the people she chooses. The integration of her Self in this way enhances both health and relationships that matter to her, including her relationship with her Self. When she loses focus, her body flashes very strong autoimmune warnings that she is dangerously close to losing her Self and her voice in her effort to maintain relationships that are not supportive of her Highest Self.

As Lila's story demonstrates, we tend to attract to our Selves the kinds of relationships that feed whatever beliefs, values, or fears we hold. Wherever you focus your attention, you will attract that kind of energy to you. Are you aware of the beliefs and intentions driving your relationships today?

When you know what qualities you want to bring to the relationship and what you require in return, your gauge for assessing actual results against your intention is clear. You can more easily detach from expectations and really see what is. Instead of wasting an enormous amount of energy and creating a significant amount of drama in your life being frustrated by or resisting what the relationship is, you can be grateful for seeing clearly what you get back for your investment of time, emotional energy, and focus in the relationship. Name what you see and do what you need to do to make your intention a reality.

You owe it to your Self to consciously and honestly assess whether the person you become in relationship with a particular idea, person, or work situation is your Best Self. If not, what kind of relationship would serve your Highest Self and what are you prepared to do to create that kind of relationship? Your choice will need to include the option of moving on, as described in Estelle's story.

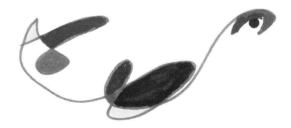

ESTELLE'S STORY OF RELATIONSHIPS

Estelle is a woman who has a strong spiritual relationship with God. She clarifies her intention and then expresses it, trusting that what comes back will fulfill her desire. Shortly after she decided, "I should have a husband," a man showed up at her front door. Her response to God was, "You're funny." She realized that if she was going to ask for help in meeting the man she would marry, she needed to be much more explicit in naming what she wanted in a relationship and in a husband. Any man that came to the door simply wouldn't do! She speaks today about how she learned to be clearer and more explicit in her desires and intention.

Her relationship with her current husband is a redefined relationship, as it was with her second husband. With her current husband, she originally chose a mature relationship fostering respect. When that relationship was insufficient to keep both of them committed to the relationship, both chose to do the necessary work individually and together to figure out how to reach a higher level of mutual vulnerability. They chose to develop ways of honoring each other's means of expression.

In an earlier incarnation of the relationship, her husband called Estelle "controlling." She recognized that he was responding to her clear relationship boundary that she would not allow her Self to be controlled by anyone else. As a result, when he told her she was controlling, she tested whether his perception might be true, reflecting a quality that limited her expression of her Best Self. Because of her clear intention, she allowed her Self to be challenged to grow more emotionally vulnerable in a relationship that would support her Best Self, and in the process, her husband's Best Self.

Together they worked on communication and an exploration of a more honest and detached perspective of what each brings to the relationship as well as what each requires to stay in it. The steps included walking away from the relationship, which gave them both the space to reflect on how much better they are as a couple than they are as individuals. She learned to be clear about what she wants from relationships. Today, when she considers the relationships in her life, Estelle is continuously asking herself how any given relationship will serve the highest in her.

She declares unequivocally that her clarity and intentionality have only gotten stronger with maturity. She continues to create the kinds of relationships that serve her, and to exit from or work to modify those that don't.

Coach's Tip: Clear intention awakens you to the need to discern healthy relationships from distractions...and shines the light for you to clearly see the truth of each one. The gap between relationships formed unconsciously using external measures and those formed consciously by listening to your intuition about which relationships support your Highest Self can be quite significant.

If you assign meaning to—frame—your relationships with work, status, money, and social identity unconsciously, you will naturally work within that frame to make the relationship work—sometimes long after you know it does not serve you. For instance, if you define your Self on some level with the amount of money you have, you develop an unconscious ego-identity tied to purchasing or having a certain house, car, or whatever in order to preserve your view of your Self. You may unconsciously frame your relationship with money as what buys you membership and social status, without seeing what it also costs you to unconsciously adopt such a frame for the relationship. Unconscious relationships often become entanglements or dependencies in which you feel trapped without realizing that the gap is between the meaning you assign the relationship and what you experience. By contrast, consciously defined relationships are easier to name for what they are. Because they are explicitly framed, you can more readily assess whether what they are and what they deliver are consistent with the meaning or frame you assign them.

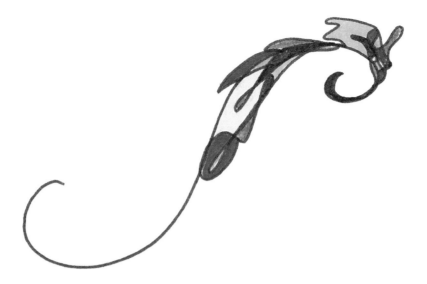

The framing of a relationship is like the frame of a barn or home. It serves to contain the relationship but it also serves to help it grow, with a kind of clarity.

EXERCISE TO TEST LEVELS OF CONSCIOUS FRAMING

This exercise is designed to help you understand the meaning you assign, perhaps unconsciously, to your relationships. That meaning becomes the frame within which you operate. To the extent you are aware of the meaning you give and the boundaries you assign to the relationship, you can make more informed decisions about the relationships that serve your Highest Self.

- Pick a relationship with a person or one with any other entity (money, job, power, status, personal identity, core belief).

- Consciously ask why this particular relationship is important in your life today. For example, if you choose your job, ask what your relationship is with that job today. Does it give you a sense of financial security or freedom? Does it help you to feel responsible or distract you from your passion? Do you derive a sense of meaning, value, or importance from your job?

- Whatever your answers, look carefully at how the meaning you give to the relationship you have with another person or entity constrains or frees you to bring your Highest Self and energy to the relationship.

Ask yourself two very critical questions:

- *Do I like who I become in the relationship?*

- *Am I aware of how the relationship plays into any of my distractions, such as—who I think I "should be" in order to be validated by others?*

Consider that the importance or meaning you may have assigned at one time to this particular relationship no longer fits what is true for you today. Notice whether you have outgrown the original frame, but have continued to try to fit who you are into it—perhaps by shrinking to only express certain parts of you.

You can do this exercise for any relationship at any point in time to assess whether the frame or meaning you assign the relationship in your life is true for you today. Use your assessments to more consciously choose to nurture those relationships that are healthy and release those that are not.

At each transition and moment of awakening, consciously choosing relationships that support your Highest Self becomes essential or you will shrink to fit into something—a relationship—you have long since outgrown. Just as a house that is comfortable for two people is too small for six, the way you defined your Self when you were disconnected from Home will need to be expanded to make space for the depth and breadth of relationships you create for your Highest Self. This does not mean that you are necessarily adding relationships. More likely, you are deepening those that are true, releasing those that are a drain, and engaging those that nurture the best in you. The conscious choices you are making about your relationships are the design decisions that ensure a thriving and beautiful garden. Now that you know how to **design for growth**, it is time to take the next step in living consciously:

Step into Your Grace

Let Grace guide your choices and Light lead the Way home to Soul's awakening.

Paula Underwood, in describing grace in the Iroquois tradition[4], spoke of the eagle and the bear. Her contention was that all animals are graceful when they are in their own environment doing what is natural for them. The majesty and grace of the eagle soaring in the sky would be hard to deny. But the eagle walking on the ground is quite awkward, hardly graceful at all. The bear, on the other hand, lumbers from side to side, interacting with all it encounters, sometimes choosing to be on four legs, other times preferring two. There is a natural and pleasing rhythm to the bear's lumbering that carries its own grace. Yet, if the bear were to try to soar like the eagle, it would be extremely awkward, not to mention completely unsuccessful in its attempts.

Grace is what you exude when, instead of trying to be something you are not, you step into all that is your Highest Self. Being true to your Highest Self and following your Inner Voice, you step into a state of ease and grace that is outwardly recognizable, although hard to describe. Like the eagle or the bear, when you wear your own skin well, you exude that grace naturally; you are "in your Grace."

Sometimes in our world today, people experience the Grace of others and try to recreate that experience by emulating others. Like asking the eagle to lumber or bear to fly, you will never find your own graceful state of being by looking outward for direction. Grace appears when you step inward to your unique essence and walk your own path. Those who walk in Grace seem to have both a stillness and vibrancy about them. There is a peacefulness that emanates from the inside. It comes from a clear Center and deep connection with their heart.

Coach's Tip: Stay connected with what is real. That is the gift of the heart to each of us. The realm of illusion is the creation of the head.

The tendency to compartmentalize life often leaves the spiritual work for times when you face a personal, often financial or health-related, crisis that rocks your sense of normalcy. You never get to live in joy and Grace by splitting life into time for reconnecting with your Center and time for everything else. Conscious living means bringing your wholeness—Highest Self—into every aspect of daily living. The opportunities for stepping into your Grace *are* those everyday activities. They are the environments to which you bring your conscious—fully awake—Self.

There is not much time for drama when you are fully alive and aware of the gifts presented in the moment. When you focus on being present—not entertaining scattered thoughts about the past or future worries—you can begin to look for how the universe is conspiring *with,* not against you to keep you on path. The beauty inherent in life itself begins to shine everywhere. And you begin to realize that experiencing beauty—in whatever way moves you to feel deeply—is an entryway to a more conscious connection with your heart and your Grace. To step into your Grace, hold the intention to:

Know beauty

Beauty is the accelerator… it is the one thing that makes me aware of my heart—it touches me to tears.

One of the main reasons it is so critical to experience life through your heart is that it is significantly more expansive than your mind. Though the heart is more powerful in its reach, the head is quicker and can distract you from the beauty around and within you. The head searches for what is missing while the heart finds the beauty and gift in whatever presents itself.

A way to bypass the head's distractions and to empower your heart to be the driver is to be fully present in every moment. You are no longer distracted by what happened in the past or might happen in the future because you are only living in the present. With an intention to be present you will find your senses heightened to the point where little things you might have missed—a stranger's smile or a warm embrace—stand out as spectacular and worthy of note. The urgency of the next e-mail or task recedes with your awareness of beauty.

Beauty is hard to write about because it is something experienced that touches the soul. Words can't recreate the experience. You know beauty when you perceive it through any or all of your senses. If you choose to be alive in every moment of your life, you are aware of the beauty in each moment and your heart is full.

If you notice beauty, you are usually compelled to stop and focus your attention on experiencing it. Typically, however, most of us are too busy trying to stay on schedule, be productive, and support our preconceived notions of how our days need to be ordered. You miss the extraordinary opportunities to reawaken from your mind-driven schedule and busyness to experience the joy of different moments in time. Beauty points to what is possible in your life, in a graceful, gentle way—no admonishing, no judgment. Being aware of beauty creates the opportunity to answer the invitation to be fully present in your heart and exhilaratingly alive in the moment.

Beauty is more about uniqueness—a moment, a shell, a sunset, a smile ...I'm coming into a period of my life where I will choose to pay attention to what nourishes, reflects beauty, brings peace, and joy.

Beauty nourishes the soul. When you fail to find the beauty in what is, whether in your Self or in others, you deny your Self the opportunity to live from the heart, in your Grace. If you know beauty, you know love. If you know beauty, you more naturally appreciate the precious miracles of life that offer themselves to you in various ways.

Take a careful look at all you do today to medicate yourself from the pain of not living from your heart, from denying your Self and others nurturance and love. What is it that you have chosen to believe that would cause you to focus on shortcomings and gaps rather than beauty and strengths in your Self and in others? Holding the intention to both seek and find beauty in your life helps you to develop an orientation to life that nourishes your garden continuously. Beauty fills up the heart and reconnects you with what it means to be completely alive, to be in a state of natural Grace. It reminds you to bring the child's sense of wonder to all you do. When you step into Grace, you remember to:

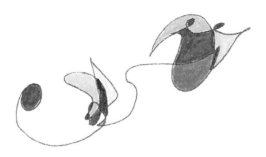

Play with life

With the delight of little things and the joy of what they bring also comes lighthearted playfulness. Suddenly things are not so serious. You can play and laugh with Life itself. Life is a dance, one that we sometimes think we are leading. Think again! It is a dance, a partnership of co-creation in each moment. To really live into your potential means to release human rules and expectations about your need to be right or to prove your worth, and choose instead to follow the Wisdom voice within. The dance is with Life itself and leading a life is following that voice, the truth of Life's process that you hold within.

The rhythm of the dance is felt in your heart and bones, not in your head. There is nothing you have to memorize or recite perfectly to be alive to life's process. There is nothing you have to figure out. The mystery of life wraps itself around you and invites you to play. Will you accept its invitation? C'mon, let go and play. The garden thrives on the spontaneous gifts of sunlight and rain. Are you as open to whatever comes your way?

What's required to be on the journey, in the dance, is commitment... Embrace Life's rhythms until they become your Nature.

There is a natural rhythm to life. It is vibrating and alive, but not frenetic. Its patterns may appear chaotic to you but that doesn't mean that they are random. It only means that you have not developed the ability to recognize or decode the underlying structures and patterns for how Life unfolds. Stay present. Watch carefully. See what happens over time. These activities can teach you how to recognize the natural rhythm of life and the underlying order that doesn't look like what the head has been taught to expect.

When you stop to watch an ant colony or look under a microscope, you experience life teeming with activity in each moment. What it means to be present and alive goes from a black and white concept to living color. Being fully awake to your own gifts and sense of lightness creates that feeling of being alive, aware of your own heart beating, aware of the beauty around and within you, attentive to the little things that bring a smile. In those moments, what matters is eminently clear. It is the simple things. It is what we have come to define as ordinary.

People with terminal illnesses often report that everything that was important to them before their illness is no longer important. The little things, that they thought were not important, really are. A beautiful sunset, a child's giggle, and the smell of fresh bread baking are magnified and raised up in their importance to feeling alive. The petty arguments about who is right and who should have been promoted shrink in importance. When you are really present in your life, you can hear the voice of intuition signaling you about what is important and what is illusion, what fills you up and what drains you. Its message is key to your stepping into Grace:

Trust your intuition

Intuition doesn't always show up at the most convenient times. It does not wait to be invited. It just shows up. Intuition is like a muscle to be exercised and nurtured. As to its power and value in life, ask your Self whether you have ever listened to your intuition and wished you had not. Then ask your Self whether you have ever failed to listen and regretted your choice. The path to a conscious life, to accessing Wisdom easily and naturally, is paved with the guidance of intuition. Intuition can help you see what you know deep in your heart, below your level of consciousness. The voice of intuition doesn't tap you on the shoulder and whisper in your ear, "Buy the blue one. It looks better on you."

Wisdom doesn't waste its time on inconsequential questions of dollars and cents. It is there to serve your Highest Self and, as long as you remember that, you can learn to understand the meaning and form of its message. Sometimes it is a feeling that comes over you and causes you to stop and notice where you are, what you are doing or about to do, and how you feel about all that. Maybe you are agreeing to do something that doesn't feel right. Your stomach feels sick at the prospect of doing the activity. But you don't want to hear this Wisdom—not now! You listen instead to external demands or to the voice in your head to override what your intuition is telling you. If you stop to pay attention to the message, there is a harvest in there for you. If you are too busy, you miss it. Here is the voice ready to serve your Best Self and help you live in graceful ease—and you are too busy? Maybe you just don't want to hear what it has to say—because deep inside you already know.

Intuition can be a fabulous wake up call. Conscious living means listening early and often. It saves a lot of trauma and drama on the back end. Its job is to help you stay on path. But then, you already know that. Intuition carries the Wisdom to guide you. Why would you ignore something that is only working on your behalf? Let intuition do its job—and let it know you are listening by following its direction. When you trust your intuition, you develop a serenity about you that comes from knowing—in every bone of your body—that you have all you need within you. You step into your Grace.

Listening to your Wisdom changes your perspective on life and on what is both real and possible. Once you know in every bone of your body what is true for you, you are at your essence, and know how it feels to be in your Grace. It is natural to not only recognize, but also appreciate, the abundance in your life and in life in general. It is about conscious awareness that there is enough for everyone—if you are open to how that looks. It is also about how consciously or unconsciously we create a world of scarcity and pain, or a world of appreciation and peace.

When you believe that there is not enough for everyone, the tendency is to guard against anyone taking your share. You become suspicious of anyone you perceive to have something you don't have, fixating on the gap rather than on what you have. People who need to compete with others for status, recognition, or power are caught in a belief that there is not enough for everyone. They are viewing the situation from the perspective of scarcity, rather than abundance. Scarcity is a learned perspective and totally incompatible with Grace. It is a creation of the mind—not the heart. Does it bring you joy and ease? Does it bring out the best in you? Why do you accept it?

EXERCISE TO TEST WHETHER YOU CHOOSE SCARCITY OR ABUNDANCE

The following prompts can help you to recognize whether you are operating from an unconscious level of fear, competition, or defensiveness, all typical indicators of scarcity.

- The next time you find yourself responding to a friend or colleague in any way that feels competitive or jealous, stop in the moment.

- Notice how you are thinking about what he or she appears to have that you don't.

- Step back to ask whether what you are thinking is what you would proudly announce to him or her that you are thinking.

- What voice is overriding your Highest Self?

- Then ask your Self what you would lose if you wished him or her well?

- How does your friend's having something you want diminish your ability to step into your potential?

Careful! Are you assuming that there is only one way for you to fulfill your deepest desires? Why? Who is talking—head or heart? Remember that scarcity lives in your head, if you let it.

If you are tied to something, such as one position to which you were both aspiring and your friend got it, step back and ask your Self why you believe this position is so critical to what you ultimately want. Perhaps your not getting the position is because it would take you off path. Or have you given up on a higher Wisdom and reverted to the illusion that your ego is more qualified to know what is best for you than your Highest Self?

- Where is your Best Self? (Hint: "absent" might be an accurate response.)

- What would happen if you just let go?

- What is the voice of intuition calling for now?

- What are you most afraid will happen if you listen?

- What perspective are you supporting—abundance or scarcity?

If you watch as your ego jumps into situations that you perceive to be win-lose, you will find ample (abundant, even) opportunity to recognize both the distractions of your mind and the callings of your heart.

Coach's Tip: When you are having trouble recognizing abundance, step back—detach. Take the time to discern where you have unconsciously detached from your heart and attached to your ego-identity.

Abundance is a perspective on life. It is a conscious choice. It is the heart's truth and the heart does not measure what the head counts as important. When you choose to design your life consciously and live into your Grace, abundance is an orientation to life that will serve you beyond your wildest dreams. It will help you recalibrate what matters in life. It will also help you to discern reality from illusion. Pay close attention because the perspective you hold on life often operates way below conscious awareness. Stay alert to your intuition and you will recognize scarcity as a human distraction, fed by external messages that produce fear and doubt. Your Highest Self knows better. When you can recognize abundance within and around you, you will naturally feel grateful for what is. In a state of Grace, you naturally:

Choose gratitude

Grace evokes gratitude and appreciation for what is. It is hard not to feel grateful when your heart is full and you are aware of how you feel. If you recognize the abundance of the universe and can look for and appreciate the—sometimes hidden—gift of any situation in your life, gratitude just flows. Choosing to see the beauty and gift in every individual and situation in which you find your Self is an orientation to life that attracts awareness of the beauty around and within you. If you cannot or will not find something to appreciate, it is because you are not ***choosing*** to appreciate something or have forgotten about having the universe as your partner in the dance of life.

Lightness and gratitude are tremendously freeing. They make it easy to appreciate the humor in your Self and in situations you create. They remind you that seriousness is a learned behavior—one that you can choose to unlearn. If you stay fully present and awake in life, you find many opportunities to experience what you encounter with lightness and humor. You might even find your Self enjoying a connection with the following message:

I live in my own little world and that's okay because they all know me here.

What fun! All that is simply is. You add the meaning. If you fail to see the opportunity to appreciate the humor, gifts, and uniqueness of any situation or individual, and focus instead on how it is different from what you thought you needed, then you are not ready to step into your Grace. When you lead with the heart, the smile of appreciation is easy. Look for the best and remain open to what might present itself. Be grateful for whatever appears. As the ancient philosopher and poet, Rumi wrote in his poem, "The Guesthouse:"[5]

This being human is a guesthouse.
Every morning a new arrival.

A joy, a depression, a meanness,
some momentary awareness comes
as an unexpected visitor.

Welcome and entertain them all!
Even if they're a crowd of sorrows,
who violently sweep your house
empty of its furniture,
still, treat each guest honorably.
He may be clearing you out
for some new delight.

The dark thought, the shame, the malice,
meet them at the door laughing,
and invite them in.

Be grateful for whoever comes,
because each has been sent
as a guide from beyond.

When you choose to respond to whatever life presents you with gratitude and appreciation, the opportunities for celebration are endless.

So, how do you help your Self shift in the moment to perceive abundance and receive whatever comes your way with gratitude? How do you stay awake to your heart and not become vulnerable to moments of overwhelming doubt? How do you recognize and follow the path of ease to your Grace? Let's return to a concept introduced earlier: noticing the difference between when you are using your energy to push something versus when you pull something towards you.

Push for clarity and pull opportunity

Push refers to the kind of energy that comes from willpower and determination. You may invoke your willpower to push your Self to do things that you find less than desirable because you determine that you need to do so for some goal you have set for your Self. For instance, let's say that you recognize where aspects of your life leave you feeling less than satisfied and searching for opportunities to make more of a difference. You push harder to make things work but the more you push, the more there is to do. You wonder why the days seem shorter, the pressures mount, and nothing seems to change. This kind of pushing is unproductive and costly. Shift your approach.

The place to push is at the front end of the process. Push your Self to clarify what your heart truly wants. Then push against your head to create the space for you to hear your heart's Wisdom—reconnect with passion and meaning.

> *Push creates the field within which illumination, Inner Voice can manifest—and be recognized. It requires discipline, time, and passion. Then, when the clarity is there, the field is set up for synchronicity to occur, at which point ease of movement is natural. Things fall in place, doors open, possibilities emerge.*

In order to push, you need a reason to want to spend the energy and life force. For example, if you want to graduate from school but do not enjoy a particular subject or doing any kind of study, you will push your Self to do the work because you care more about graduating than about enjoying what you need to do in the immediate moment to get there. If you want to make it to the top of an organization, you may push your Self to work on projects or in locations that you do not really want in order to be qualified for promotion. Push energy is forceful and works against something. It involves resisting some other force.

If you do not push to create the space to hear your heart, your lack of clarity sets you up to entertain doubt and fear when social convention, popular messages, or the distractions of your mind contradict your vague sense of what you want. ***Your lack of clarity about what you really want***—not how you think it must look or when you want it to happen—leads you to think that if you don't take control, your life will never turn out as you want it to be. You end up spending your time and energy resisting what happens in your life, and correcting situations to be what you think you want them to be.

If you look back on your life, I suspect that you will find many examples of energy spent pushing ***how*** when what actually happened got you to where you needed to be anyway. Applying to colleges and believing that only a certain one would make you happy and then going somewhere else—for whatever reason—and having that experience be exactly what you needed is one example. The same thing happens when you desperately want one particular job, don't get it, and find out later that not getting the one you wanted served you well. The list goes on.

> *The push/pull aspect of life needs to be reframed. The push requires energy in the form of focus, clarity, and stillness. It is not the step that follows getting clear. It's the step to clarity...(once clear) it's time to pull, meaning respond to all that is ... by getting behind it and simply supporting all that wants to be. We are doing it all backwards!*

Life does not need to be so difficult. As the quote above indicates, we are going about it backwards. The resistance needs to be at the front end. Resist the distractions of your mind. Resist the need for approval and acceptance. Push inward and hear what your heart wants deeply. Resist the head's voice that creating time for your Self is selfish or costly, because someone else who wants your time and attention is not getting it. Push for what you know is necessary for you to serve your highest potential, your greatest version of living your purpose.

If you push at the beginning of anything for whatever time and space is necessary to be absolutely clear about your intention and desire, you are prepared to recognize all of the support that comes your way to make it happen. Being fully present to recognize the realm of possibilities that suddenly emerge, pop into your life—seemingly from nowhere—is the energy of **pull**. For example, if you decide to be your Best Self in all contexts and that Best Self loves a good laugh, then you will know to accept invitations to participate in events or with particular people that make it easy for you to laugh and enjoy yourself, and reject those that don't.

When you are very clear about the person you choose to be and what ultimately matters in your life, you are less tied to the rules of social convention and approval. You are less inclined to use your energy to hold onto things and people that are not aligned with your path. You can now devote your attention to watching and listening for what comes your way and pulling from those possibilities the ones that match who you want to be and what you seek to create. You experience the abundance of possibilities from which to choose. Instead of pushing your way through life, you are more relaxed and peaceful, alert to what is happening and ready to pull anything that comes your way that supports your path. Gratitude fills your approach to life and Grace leads the way. You are naturally being and supporting your Highest Self.

TUNE-UP EXERCISE IN CONSCIOUS CHOICE

To test whether you have pushed to create enough clarity at your Center to make very conscious choices, carefully observe your behavior. What is your response to each of the following questions? Pay attention to how your body feels as you answer each of the questions.

- Do you offer "little white lies" or long explanations when you decline requests or invitations? Why?

- Are you taking care of others? Are you doing their work for them?

- Is your ego-identity challenged because you want to be seen as nice?

- Are you declining requests or invitations that you do not want to be accepting? If not, why not?

- To which voices are you giving more power than to the voice of your heart?

- When the voices pop into your head to question decisions you have already made, do you dismiss the voices to stay present, or do you feed on their seduction to engage guilt or doubt?

- How clear are you about the person you choose to be in your life and what kind of impact or legacy you wish to leave?

Are you committed enough to a life of meaning that you will push your Self to get clear? If so, when you are finished, repeat this exercise—several times! If not, you are abandoning your Highest Self and your life's path in favor of an unconscious existence.

Stepping into your Grace is stepping into the fullness of your potential. It is rooted in your deep connection to all that is highest in who you are at your Center. This connection feeds your desire to bring all of you—not just the pieces validated in certain contexts or by particular people—into full expression in your life. In so doing, you achieve the ability to function in many contexts and relationships without compromising your integrity—your wholeness. Contrary to popular belief, wholeness is not achieved by focusing on finding balance among the different aspects of your Self.

> *Balance is a by-product of integration (not an end unto itself). When balance is the focus, fragmentation and separateness are the means.*

When you focus on balance, you unwittingly fragment your life further, trying to figure out which part of you can show up in which relationships and situations. Does the playful one with a slight edge not show up at work because someone else might not approve? Does the nice you shut down your voice with friends and family who don't deal with conflict? If you preserve the integrity and wholeness of your Highest Self, all of you can live a life of Grace.

> *Be at Home in your Heart...It's a deep listening to what stirs or moves the heart that guides activity.*

You have stepped into your Grace by knowing beauty, playing with life, trusting the Wisdom of your intuition, and choosing to respond to all life brings with gratitude. By deeply connecting with your heart in the context of your daily living, you are prepared to bring the voice of clarity to an unconscious world of external noise. Now that you know how to ***step into your Grace***, the next step in designing your Self for conscious living is to:

Speak from Your Heart

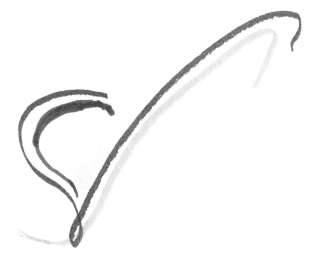

Only when you are deeply connected to your heart can you know its desires. When you are fully present and able to hear your Inner Voice, you are able to:

Consciously know your intention

Whether you are conscious or unconscious, clear or unclear, you are attracting people and situations to you all the time. Intention is a magnet that shapes energy. If you want to attract something different from what you have been attracting, then it is time to check your intention. When you enter a meeting, conversation, or any situation, do you know explicitly what you want from it and what you choose to contribute? What is your intention for how you will be, what you will and will not bring to the situation, and what you require in return? This is not about engineering every situation and relationship in which you participate. It is being clear about what your heart wants. Maybe it is just to be included in whatever happens. Maybe it's more.

When you are in the realm of passions and desires, you are out of your mind. Your mind only thinks it knows what you want. Your heart and soul really do have the key to what brings you joy, what nourishes your soul right to its core, what speaks to whatever is highest in you—and, indeed, to all of humanity. When your heart is clear and you listen, your head knows how to support the intention you hold. When Inner Wisdom speaks, are you willing to listen?

CONSCIOUS INTENTION EXERCISE

Clarifying your intention involves separating your heart's desires from fears, doubts, and the unconscious need for control. The next time you have a scheduled meeting or a planned conversation with someone in particular, take a few quiet moments prior to the conversation to ask your Self:

What results do I want from the conversation?

Beware of any answers that detail specific behaviors you want from other people.

- If you want Joe to change his mind as a result of a meeting you have, recognize that you are setting yourself up for failure. You are caught in the "I'm right and you just don't get it" mentality.

- If you want Joe to hear your point of view, that is a very different intention from expecting him to respond in a certain way. Consider what you want Joe to understand of your perspective and whether you are truly willing to understand Joe's thinking.

- If you are not willing to hear his perspective, why are you engaging him in conversation? Remember that the choice to respond to anyone and to any situation in any particular way lives within each of us.

When you hold specific outcomes for other people, it just means that you haven't gone deep enough into your heart to find out what you truly want. Your head may be interfering with your connection to your heart. Specific outcomes are usually what your head has convinced you will get you whatever you really want.

Sit with the question of why you care how the other person responds. That way you can surface your reasoning and separate it from what you truly want. Then ask your Self the following question:

Who is the person I choose to be in this conversation?

If you are meeting with someone in whose presence you get nervous and forget what you want to say:

- Take some time to disconnect from what you think she or he thinks of you.

- Remember why you are having the conversation in the first place.

- Come back to the question of the person you are when you are at your best, and consciously choose to bring that person to the conversation.

You can practice asking your Self the two critical questions in any context, until it becomes second nature for you to connect with your heart and know your deepest intention. It will save you a lot of energy and pushing in the long run.

Clear intention to remain true to what you most enjoy about your Self and to stay in your heart can help you to take things less personally. The important step here is that you are very clear about who you will be in that conversation—because that will help you listen to Wisdom that directs you when to respond and when to ask for more time because something does not feel right.

Coach's Tip: If you hold the conscious intention to be your Highest Self, you create the opportunity to attract the same in others. Listen to your heart for instructions about what to do and what not do in the moment.

Conscious living means paying attention to your heart. It means being so present that you notice—without analyzing—every thought as it pops into your head. It means stopping to ask your Self whether following any particular thought leads you to be your very Best Self or distracts you from your wisdom. Holding a clear intention to bring out only the best in you means that you are open to pull towards you any of a number of possible responses to any situation. It makes it easier for you to:

Speak your truth

No matter where you find your Self today, the ability to communicate with other people in ways that are true to who you are and respectful of others' Highest Selves is essential. When you speak from your heart, you speak from truth and Wisdom. The rest falls into place. You do not need to engineer messages and rehearse them in your head. Much less effort is required. Just hold the intention and listen for instructions. Try it. You will find that it will only work when you stay connected to your heart and hold the clear intention that whatever serves your truth you will have. Trust in the wisdom of your own truth to express your Highest Self and let go of whether others will be comfortable with what you have to say.

> *Putting color and daring back in my life are critical. They are life supports for me. Yet I have toned down my emotional responses, colors, and who knows what else so as to conform, not offend.*

It is not uncommon to shut down your voice, to not express what you know to be true, and to even doubt what you believe to be true when it goes against conventional wisdom. Unless your intention to operate from truth exceeds your desire to fit in, you will not be inclined to bring your full voice to the situation or relationship. With continued practice in this vein, you can easily become a shell of your Highest Self, uncomfortable expressing your Self, if you even remember who she or he is. The focus of your energy is diverted to meet others' expectations of you. Such a diversion is exhausting and not in service of the greater good. Your Wisdom is missing in action from a world that needs it.

When you find your Self in doubt and muffling your voice, ask your Self the question a wise woman once asked me:

> *Who would you be, if you were one hundred times bolder?*

Another wise woman, Marianne Williamson,[6] offers her perspective on the importance of boldly stepping into the fullest expression of your Self and voice in the following way:

...Your playing small doesn't serve the world.
There is nothing enlightened about shrinking
so that others won't feel insecure around you.
... as we let our light shine: we consciously
give others permission to do the same.

Desire for the truth serves not only your individual expression of your Best Self. It also serves the greater good, as others allow themselves to be more aware of their gifts. If they are not ready, at least you will know that, and you can make a choice about with whom and how you choose to invest your time and energy. You can continue to delve more deeply into the essence of your Self and to express your voice, or you can cede the floor to those who do not want to hear or are afraid of your clarity. Which do you choose in your thoughts and actions today?

Coach's Tip: The real key to communicating truthfully and in ways that honor who you are is more about clarity of intention and ability to hear your Inner Wisdom than anything else.

Watch carefully for the tricky voice in your head that tells you that others know more. Test what they claim to know against your heart, even when what your heart tells you differs from conventional wisdom. You may find that the practical or "proven" advice is not the one that is true for you. When you begin to listen to your own truth, you may find your Self at odds with others who do not want you to be following any truth but the one they hold. That knowledge may begin to signal you about where you want to invest your energy and time. It may be time to assess the cost of belonging with these others, and the nature and meaning of these relationships in your life.

FINE TUNING EXERCISE

This exercise is designed to help you recognize how easily you shift from hearing your own truth to listening to and being swept up by external voices.

- Try singing any song in rounds with a few friends.

Singing in rounds means that each of you sings the same thing but at different times, always overlapping each other. One commonly used song for this exercise is "Row, Row, Row Your Boat." There are many others. You can use any simple song.

- Notice how, over time, you either continue to hold your own melody and words, or you end up singing the words and melody of someone else whose voice may be stronger or louder than yours.

This little reminder can help you attune your awareness to how well you are listening to your own voice, hearing your own Wisdom—and holding the intention to do so when in the presence of other voices and opinions.

An alternative to singing in rounds is to:

- Practice singing one song while a different song is playing in the background.

- Once you pay attention to the background music, notice how long it takes for you to begin singing your own song off key or to forget the words of your song.

If you try this often, you will be able to quickly remind your Self what it takes to be able to hear your voice and Wisdom when you are surrounded by other distractions.

There are contexts and groups of people—families, nations, religions—with very clear boundaries for membership and success. If your work in the world or what fills you is tied to being a part of these contexts, then being able to detach and hear Wisdom about the environment and people is critical. Estelle's story reflects her experience in dealing with membership in certain segments of society, and the line she draws to stay true to her own Wisdom when considering the value of belonging.

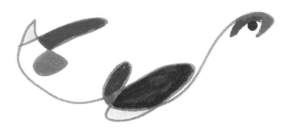

ESTELLE'S STORY OF VOICE

A strong leader in the African American community, Estelle has always sensed the strong influence of her identity as an African American and as a woman on both her sense of Self and her self esteem. Growing up, she was not given permission to speak up, to voice her views. Her parents were leaders in a fundamentalist church and she was clearly shown that there was a place for little girls.

Along the way, in her own young adult years, she developed a political consciousness about what Black families, and especially Black men, need in order to be heard and for their personhood to be supported. She identified very clearly what she believed she needed to do, say, and be to serve what she identified as the "Black man's need to carry his yoke on the job."

She perceived that it was critical for women to accommodate these men and their burden so she shut down her voice. But that only lasted for so long. She recognized that there was a line that she was not willing to cross. Estelle chose, at a point in time, that she was not going to own the Black man's place. This clear intention inspired and required her to spend time figuring out exactly where the line was if she chose not to accept his burden. She was very clear that she would always have a piece of her Self left for her at the end of the day. She became very conscious of the line and knows exactly where it is today. She will leave a relationship before she will cross that line.

Never one to be lost in a crowd, this woman has always carried herself with distinct presence, alternatively intimidating and inspiring others. In the work context, she has been told that she, "walks in the room in charge." It is a way of carrying her Self. Each of her male mentors has said the same thing. She also recognizes that she is very sexy, and has consciously chosen to turn it off at work to avoid being misunderstood or perceived as threatening by others.

An extremely competent leader and manager, she modulates not only what she says but also the delivery of her message in order to be heard and not threaten those with whom she needs to partner to succeed. As she learned how to be comfortable with her Self, she became less rebellious, and more comfortable with how to use her voice. She is not abandoning who she is. Rather she has figured out what to tone down to be true to her Self and bring her best gifts to bear. She says that the way she thinks about it is the same way she "thinks about when to turn the light on." And that is, "only when the room needs to be illuminated."

As Estelle continues to step into increasingly higher consciousness and the realization of her gifts, she retains the learner's stance in different contexts. Today she is very conscious of whether the other person is ready to receive her message. The challenge she is working on now is walking the line of how to be truthful in a way that does not turn away those whom she seeks to reach and remain in relationship with on a much broader scale, while being true to her Highest Self. She continues to clarify just where that line is for her.

You will need to determine where your line is. As you do so, hold the intention not only to bring out the best in you, but also to help others rise to their potential. When you hold this intention, how to accomplish your goal becomes clear. Your intention is not about who you want someone else in the relationship to be, or how you want another to behave. It is not about changing outside things. It is only about changing the person you are in relationships with other people, situations, beliefs and ideas.

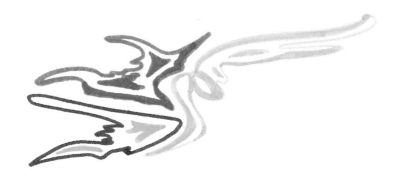

On the journey to greater consciousness, you learn to recognize the value of lighting the way for others on the journey. You also feel gratitude for others who do the same. The whole process shifts your focus to finding your own light and sharing it with others so they can also find their own. There is no competition among sojourners. Being your best doesn't require that someone else be "less than." What would be the point? You recognize that anyone who chooses to live a more conscious life serves all who choose the same. The focus is on finding the best in everyone and working to make everyone shine through their unique gifts and strengths—to help them live into their life's purpose and highest potential.

We seem most able to recognize the truth of this mindset when there is a crisis and ego identity is put aside to help those in need. Stripped of title, office, and status, we step in to work together to help others survive a crisis, whether it is a tsunami, an earthquake, or a fire. It is time to take this natural way of operating and move it from the realm of surviving to the realm of thriving. To help others thrive, you can extend a hand and not worry about whether you are the most qualified. See what's called for. Offer what you have to give. Create a context where your Best Self awakens the Best Self in others. Make room for roles to change as needs and resources change.

One story comes from a worker who has developed his own values quite consciously, and who speaks honestly and openly about his choices when asked. He doesn't always offer them without prompting, although he is very generous when he believes that what he knows could help another in a similar situation. One of his gifts is a thoughtful and reflective manner of sharing his experiences.

In one particular setting where a group of colleagues was developing their ability to work as a team, a new member of the group expressed disappointment at not ever having been formally welcomed by the team. Several colleagues questioned this worker because they felt that they had been treating him as if he had always been a member. But this one worker acknowledged the situation and offered honestly that he had not welcomed the new person to the team because he hadn't been ready to welcome him. He went on to say that he was now ready to welcome the new member and did so.

Others in the group were shocked by his directness and honesty. No one questioned his intent, including the new member who promptly thanked him. It was a fascinating situation. The behaviors expressed offered a perfect illustration of what happens when your intent is pure and comes from love. The worker not only brought out his Best Self but also enabled the group to reach a higher level of trust and openness where all of their individual gifts could shine.

This situation illustrates how when you walk in light and speak from truth and love, the intention is recognized, even if the words are not exactly what others are ready for or want to hear. If you look honestly within your Self, you will probably recognize a willingness to make space for others who may be a bit awkward in what they are trying to express, when you know that their intent is pure. Instead of resisting these messages, you are naturally drawn to support or help.

We have all been in situations where we and other people have not felt safe in expressing what we know or feel. Sometimes when you serve your Highest Self in a way that brings out the best in others, you may pause and reflect before voicing your perspective. There will be other times when your heart is so clear that you speak before you even think about your words, and what you say is absolutely what is needed to be said at the time, as in the situation described above.

To support the best in everyone, you need only come from love. Once your intention is grounded in love, it is easy and natural to express honesty with the sensitivity and sensibility that help others appreciate your honesty. This is a simple concept, but a difficult stance if you haven't done the in-dwelling to detach from unconscious ego needs and power games.

Some people who are unconsciously driven by their own ego insecurities may be unwilling to acknowledge that they don't really know what is in their heart. They spend an enormous amount of energy trying to prove their own view is right. If you respond to them from your head, they are likely to escalate the need to prove their point. The conversation gets heated and Best Selves disappear. What works instead is to remain centered in love and true to your Best Self. Trust your heart to know if silence or specific words feel right. Others may not know what to do with you in that moment, but you will have provided some light for them to either rise to the occasion and shine, or to reflect on at a later point. It is probably worth a reminder that when you speak from love you may wish the best for another, but it does not mean that you hold a particular outcome for someone else. Holding a particular outcome in mind for someone else attracts resistance and limits your own ability to be true to your Highest Self.

When you are unaware of your ego's desire to perform and shine, you may find your Self preoccupied with having the exact right words. You may get caught in a web of personal performance, attempting to shine above the rest or prove your Self most worthy, competent, or intelligent. If you are worried about performing well, you are in your head and not present to guidance from your heart. You are playing an ego role, rather than consciously choosing what supports the Best in you. Every moment of every day is an opportunity to reflect, before responding, on what qualities you bring when you speak from your heart with clear intention to serve your Highest Self and the best in others.

When I was invited to speak at my father's sixtieth high school reunion, I was honored and wanted to be able to honor my Dad by whatever I said. I struggled to find something worthy to say to a generation whom I admire and respect, and who have thirty more years of life experience than I do. It took a fair amount of reflection to recognize that my speaking wasn't about me. It was about serving a group for whom I have the utmost admiration, at a time in their lives when recognition is not so often accorded in our youth-centric society. Once my intention was clear, love was the only lens through which my words would be filtered. Frankly, I don't remember what I said. I only know that in looking out at the group gathered, I felt nothing but love and gratitude for the opportunity to thank them for all they have done. Their gifts became the focus. My gift was to remind them of theirs.

Stay centered when others don't respond from love

Consider the challenges of being in full voice when those around you not only have no capacity to hear or receive your message, but also appear to intend you harm. Your ability to detach from their negative focus and check your body for guidance is a good place to start. Your intuition will signal you whether the situation and the response you are planning will put you in harm's way or not. Assuming that you are in no serious physical danger, your ability to stay connected with your heart grounds you in the moment. You can separate others' unconsciousness and harmful wishes from your Self and see the situation with a detached perspective. For instance, if you are delivering a difficult message, you may be confronted with anger or particularly vicious accusations. If you stay centered, you can appreciate the fear behind the anger and attacks. This, in turn, allows you to create the context for others to appreciate your calmness without being defensive. If you stay in your own light and don't resist the situation or messages you hear from others, you may create the opportunity to reframe the situation in a way that clearly communicates the integrity of your Best Self.

> Be in the energy but separated from it. It will dissipate if you look directly at it...Stay in the Light. Don't resist. Don't give in. Practice standing strong and letting what needs to fall away do so.

To respond as described you need to be centered in who you are at your essence. Once centered in your heart and clear about your intention, you have the opportunity to stand tall and face the anger or intended threats in a way that allows you to detach from the emotion and hear the words. The ability to detach in those moments where others may be less aware of the anger with which they speak creates an opportunity to respond thoughtfully so that they feel heard, while at the same time not internalizing the anger or heat of the situation.

In the context of being heard, often others will retract the anger. I have been in situations where a great deal of heat, anger, or frustration was directed at me by others who perceived that I was having influence they did not want me to have. By staying in the situation, detaching from attacks, and listening for what was behind the message, I had the opportunity to ask questions to better understand the true source of the speakers' frustration or anger. After they calmed down, people offered that, "It really wasn't about you personally." People who are caught in unconscious roles or ego identities are sometimes prone to unconscious emotional outbursts. These outbursts may be made without awareness of the full impact of the words and force on others. You can either sink to that level of awareness and retaliate, or help raise the level for all to operate more consciously.

Choosing to only engage in situations and relationships in ways that support your Best Self certainly colors how and whether you will choose to respond to others who direct their anger and negativity at you. It will also affect how you respond to people who direct anger and frustration indiscriminately, and you happen to be in their path. If responding in a particular way helps you express your Highest Self, regardless of immediate reaction from others, you are most likely speaking from the heart and the situation or relationship is on path for you. If it continues to draw you away from your Center and into the heat of the conversation and your ego identity, perhaps the relationship is not one that serves your Best Self. Seek opportunities elsewhere!

Coach's Tip: When you choose to step into your Grace and speak from your heart, you live into your unique life purpose.

Who you are as your Highest Self, what unique gifts and qualities characterize your Best Self, and what focus of energy inspires and fills your heart are all about purpose. Living purposefully brings meaning and a sense of fulfillment, while it tickles your soul. Discovering what is on purpose for you and what qualities describe your Highest Self requires no figuring out. It requires no outside research. It does take dispassionately observing your choices and results and testing whether they touch your heart and fill you up. When you are on purpose, it is natural to speak from the heart.

Remember that the journey to higher consciousness does not carry with it a sword for bashing those who are not ready to go. Self-righteous responses that demand that workplaces and relationships change to suit your journey or passion need to be tempered by remembering that any group or relationship—such as, with a workplace—has rules for membership. If you like them and they serve your purpose, stay. If not, recognize that you may need to change or leave. The option that works for you depends on what will support your life's purpose, and reconnect you with your passion and heart. The decision to stay in a relationship, including working in a particular place, is a choice of conscious membership. The rules for membership are the price you pay to play—to belong. What allows you to experience what you seek from the relationship and serve your purpose in life is the fourth and last step in consciously living—by design:

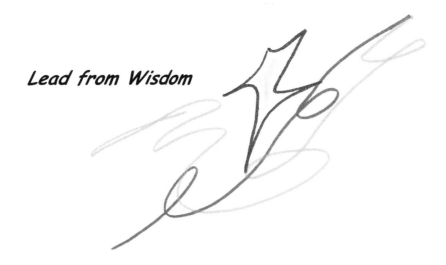

Lead from Wisdom

What does it mean to lead from Wisdom? It means being aware of and detached from what is happening in the moment at the same time as you are deeply connected to your Highest Self. It means *following the voice of your heart in choosing how and who you will be in every present moment.* It is about continuously taking your pulse. What is happening in this moment? How do I choose to be? What response is the voice of my Highest Self? In order to follow your Wisdom, you have to listen *for* it and *to* it. Just as when you take your own pulse, you have to stop, focus on what you are doing, and then wait to feel the heartbeat. When you go inward—in-dwelling—you prepare the soil to receive Wisdom. When you bring that Wisdom to your everyday life—Away—you:

Consciously and continuously tend your garden

In your choice to live the conscious life—to lead from Wisdom, the soil of your garden needs continuous nourishment from *four essential nutrients: clarity, compassion, courage, and faith.*

Clarity

Clarity is an incredibly powerful asset, one that requires vigilant attention. Too often we do not take the time to be clear about what we want from our actions before we take the action. As a result, life becomes a series of increased distractions until you lose touch with who you choose to be and what you choose to create with your life.

From the earlier discussions of push versus pull, you know that in the face of external demands, social pressure to conform, and unconscious identity with the roles you perform, you have to push against distractions to create the space to hear your heart. By pushing for space, you create the intention to listen to your heart—to listen *for* Wisdom. Clarity is the result of also listening *to* the Wisdom of your heart.

Coach's Tip: You have to be committed to creating the space in your life in order to hear the Inner Voice that provides the clarity you seek.

When you create the space and time to be clear about your intention, you choose more consciously where to invest your time and energy. You also become very clear about what you want in return for your investment. Clarity gives you the courage to say "no" when that is what is needed to serve your Best Self. When you are clear about what is important to you, what you perceive as a risk is very different from what social convention might tell you.

...wanting to live an inspired life and taking whatever turns are needed to be true to that value

Imagine that the above statement is true for you. If it were, you would not be afraid of what might occur around the bend. The deep desire to live an inspired life would bring with it a commitment to continually ask whether a particular relationship or decision leads towards or away from inspiration. Choosing something because it is safe or predictable would be more of a risk to living the life that you want than going out on a limb that inspires new growth. Risks are only defined in the context of the clarity of your heart's desires. Anything less than clarity about heart's desire to be your Highest Self and live your passion produces a very risky path in terms of your life's purpose. From the vantage point of social convention, however, the path appears to be safer and more secure when you follow your head because that is the escape route being chosen by so many others. Only in the context of clarity is the risk-benefit relationship defined in a meaningful way for each individual. You will need to be alert, present, and conscious of what moves your heart to hear the Wisdom about risky versus healthy choices for a purposeful life.

Getting clear is a process, a series of choices that support illumination and an enlightened perspective. In essence, getting clear is a continuous journey Home to connect and reconnect with what is true at your Center. Living consciously every day means that you are pausing to reflect on the choices you are considering, listening for your body's response, and then following the Wisdom within. In-dwelling becomes an ongoing practice—not an event that you engaged once in your life when things weren't going very well. The soil needs to be fed with the essential nutrients and the soul nurtured continuously to support the magnificence of a life lived consciously.

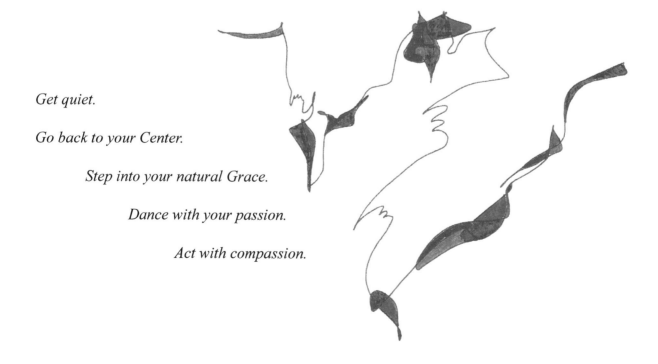

Get quiet.

Go back to your Center.

Step into your natural Grace.

Dance with your passion.

Act with compassion.

Compassion

The path to a more conscious existence is available to all who choose to engage it. It neither requires that everyone participate nor prevents anyone from accepting the invitation. The path appears scary to some, forbidden to others, and welcoming to others. The last group will go on the journey with little encouragement. If you choose to go, go gently and without judgment. Doing so allows others who are tentative or resistant sojourners to gracefully change their minds, and not have to worry about losing face, if and when they want to start along the path at a later time. Responding with compassion, rather than judgment creates openings for people to change, to step up, or to see situations and themselves differently. Judgments tend to foster resistance and defensiveness because they tap into unconscious fears and distractions about being good enough and not fulfilling others' expectations. Far more is achieved by creating "graceful openings."

Creating graceful openings means that you are never judging another for her or his choice to hesitate or not get on path early on. Rather you create an atmosphere that is welcoming, doesn't ask a thousand questions when another chooses to take a step, and embraces each step taken with love. No matter how many times someone—including you—loses the way, abandons the path, or reengages, you are only paying attention to encouraging and welcoming those conscious choices to get back to purpose and Best Self. Some will want to see how the path has served others they know and respect before taking their own steps. They are not prepared to lead but they may choose to get on their own paths by accessing graceful openings left by others who are leading the way. Gentle compassion and appreciation, for whoever shows up at whatever points, create a field of receptivity that supports the conscious journey. Compassion envelops all, including your Self, in a loving embrace that supports growth. Compassion is a reaching out, a welcoming that you extend to your Self and others. You know in your heart that we are all on a journey where what one learns can help everyone else.

Coach's Tip: Compassion is essential to living in Grace.

Compassion is easier for people who approach life from abundance, rather than from a scarcity mentality. By recognizing that there is enough for everyone if you are not attached to exactly how that looks, you are more willing to share resources and appreciate where another is on the journey. You understand that it is not your job to change anyone else. You come to recognize that most people are doing the best they can with where they are in their lives at any given time. Empathy and appreciation are natural states. The need to compete for resources is gone. Growth and increased opportunities to flourish are fostered. Choosing to respond to people and situations with compassion opens you to seeing and appreciating the gifts of any situation or individual's actions, rather than resisting because they are different from what you might have expected or thought you needed. Anger and frustration dissipate. Patience, understanding, and love grow.

> *I'm surprised sometimes at how frustrated or angry I can get, allowing myself to be threatened by others' behaviors that I perceive to reflect on me or make me look bad. Such a ridiculous concept when I see it on paper. But unless I am clear and listen to my truth and then detach from the situation, I can get stuck. I'm learning to recognize that part of me, and be less judgmental.*

Compassion and gentleness need to be turned inward, as well as outward. Many people are harder on themselves than they would ever be on anyone else. Why? How does that harshness foster your Highest Self and Wisdom? How does it support appreciating your inner beauty and unique gifts? What end is it serving? Compassion brings a needed gentleness to life, whether reflected inward on your Self or extended outward to others. It is a natural by-product of being in your Grace and an essential nutrient in leading from Wisdom. When you nurture your soul with compassion, you will find it much easier to lead from courage.

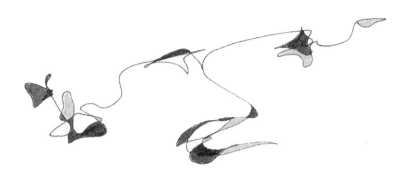

Courage

It takes some courage to let go of what's known to step into the unknown. I don't know the timing. I don't know what form my work will take.

Today we have become rather complacent, choosing immediate comfort and validation over inspired and passionate lives. We often measure success in dollars, things, and social status rather than in lives impacted, differences made, and potential realized. Yet, many people today are searching. We are beginning to awaken to that underlying drive for meaning and to listen for the Wisdom within. The environment today is ripe—or perhaps, begs—for courageous decisions to be made, both individually and collectively.

Clarity is what allows you to more easily be true to your Highest Self. Courage moves you from a clear picture of who you choose to be and what you want to create with your life to making the choices that support that clear picture. Courageous choices are ones that take you past your comfort zone on one hand, and directly into your Highest Self on the other. Courage is like intuition, a capacity to which all have access and one that gets much easier to access with practice. It is possible that after several courageous choices, you will not even think of your choices as courageous—only as whatever is required to be your Best Self, following the Wisdom of your path.

Compassion and courage go hand in hand. The integrity of who you are as your Best Self may have been neglected through outward focus on pleasing others and choices made to fit into organizations or groups whose membership you have valued. Compassion for Self and the choices you have made, coupled with the commitment to lead from your Highest Self, makes courageous decisions easier. Gentleness, rather than harsh judgment and fear of punishment, makes it easier to summon courage. With more courageous choices you may find yourself more empathic towards people who limit their own potential and are having difficulty summoning the courage to lead from Wisdom. Extending compassion can help them to summon the courage they need on their journey as well.

A wonderful example comes from an intact group whose work includes helping each other to step more boldly into their Best Selves. They probably would not have sought each other out as friends, but they have learned to work together to get great results. Over time, each of the members has developed his or her style of leading in ways that respect the different values and preferences of the other members.

In one particular case, a group member, who had traditionally taken the role of accommodator, summoned the courage to declare what she wanted to do prior to hearing others' preferences. Initially, she appeared to do so without much regard for what others wanted or needed, as she blurted out her positions. As she was learning to express her opinions, two others in the group stepped up to congratulate her for being clear about what she wanted. They chose to support her courage, while helping her to speak her truth in ways that also supported the others' needs in the group. They gently reminded her and the group of their commitment to foster their Best Selves. In so doing they reiterated the group norms for speaking honestly—and with compassion for others in the group. The group developed a way of testing each other, while welcoming diversity of perspective in the group. The former accommodator became a more vocal member of the group and the group learned how to help her test whether she is reacting from her head or living courageously from her heart—leading from Wisdom.

What is it that makes the courageous choice the easier path? Absolute clarity and commitment to purpose and to Best Self are essential for engaging the courageous choices that are not common in today's world. In the early stages of the journey, it is hardest to act with courage because you have very little experience with a new way and the power of convention is always a tempting distraction. You may need additional support—another nutrient for the soil—when unlearning old ways and breaking out of ways you distract your Self from your truth. When the old ways no longer work and the new path is not yet clear, it is time for faith.

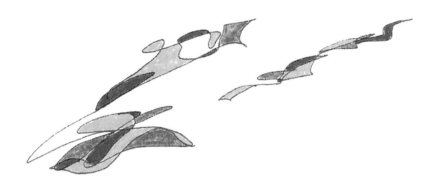

Faith

We tend to speak of faith when things are going well. But faith is about knowing in every cell of your body that something that you cannot see or demonstrate concretely in physical terms is true. That truth provides clarity in times of doubt. Faith in a guiding hand, Life itself, or Divine Wisdom provides the context for perceiving something to be supportive that you might not otherwise have recognized as such. For instance, if you believe there is a grand plan and that whatever happens is supporting both your unique path and a greater good, then you might persuade yourself to consider something like a relationship's apparent downturn or job loss as clearing the way for you to focus on something more critical to your purpose. Rather than being susceptible to fear and doubt, you would be centered in faith and able to recognize the Wisdom that guides you forward. Faith in something bigger than your mind supports detachment from a specific outcome and from specific expectations about timing. It encourages openness to seeing other possibilities.

Here is an example from my own life where faith in Divine timing and Wisdom was tested. My business partner and I had talked of opening an institute for people to disconnect from busy lives and reconnect with their Center. We found a fabulous site—twenty acres of rolling pasture, with an old barn, homestead, and third structure. Even though we had talked about being near the water, this bucolic setting seemed perfect. It needed a lot of work, but the price was right and it was gorgeous. On the day we had to submit our bid, we were under a tight deadline. As I typed away on the computer, we finished, with minutes to spare, and hit the print button. The printer, which had been working perfectly the day before, would not print. We tried everything. Finally, exasperated, I decided to write the offer out by hand. Once I began, the printer started. It printed the first page and stopped. We tried again. Again when I overrode the printer's "refusal" to get the job done for us, it successfully printed the second page.

You will probably not be surprised to learn that the bid was acceptable to the prospective sellers but the terms were not. In the long run, we walked away from the property—laughing at the printer's signal that might have saved us some time—if we had been willing to listen. But the message was bigger. As it turns out, we refined our entire picture of what the institute could be and do. When we did, we realized that what we really wanted was a gathering place that anyone in the community could access. We continued to refine the concept until we ended up focusing on a portion of what was to be in the institute—a tea shop that sells art, encourages new artists by showing their work, and partners with communities to create a gathering place for conversation and workshops. But the story doesn't end here.

We found the "ideal" spot several times! Each time, there was a voice encouraging us to choose a particular location that was being developed and wouldn't be ready for another year or two. We refused and went after—and got close each time to—two other locations. Each time, something—finances or issues with sellers—stopped us. We stood back. At a time when we had just about put the tea shop concept on the back burner, the property we had been ignoring or resisting was ready. It was smaller than we thought we needed it to be. Other things were also different. But, once we said, "yes" to the new location, financing opened up, and people came out of the woodwork to encourage, support, and help make the whole thing happen.

We had to wait for the building to be built. We had to continually test our intention—what to hold close and what to release to be true to the dream. The timing was not what we had expected, but in retrospect, we both can see where everything that needed to be lined up to support our vision happened—according to a plan wiser than our own. We needed to stay open to how our dream could happen.

Some people today are so afraid of making a mistake that they become paralyzed. They are afraid to try something without knowing exactly where it will lead or exactly what might happen. They stay in dead-end relationships of every kind, calculating the cost of making new friends, learning a new job, having to move, or being disapproved of by others whom they admire without calculating the cost of not following their heart. Such choices are not of faith. They are of fear.

Coach's Tip: Fear disconnects the power cord to the heart and gives power to doubt and outside forces. Faith reconnects the power cord to the heart and disables doubt and fear.

Clarity reminds you to consciously choose faith when the temptations of doubt or fear present themselves. Faith and compassion make it easier to laugh at your Self. They encourage you to appreciate wherever you are and to gently move to wherever your Best Self is nurtured. Faith and clarity help you to summon the courage to stand firmly where needed and pull from Wisdom all that truly supports your intention.

HEAVY REMINDERS EXERCISE

If you want to be lighthearted and free, this exercise can help you shine the light on where you are undermining your ability to do so.

The next time you find your Self doubting what your heart tells you to do:

- Go to the yard or street and pick up a few rocks. They need to be relatively substantial in size—bigger than pebbles and small enough for you to carry in one hand.

- Bring them back inside.

- Sit with the doubt until you can recognize the belief or fear that you are holding.

- If you know, for example, that you hold your Self back from trying something you want to try because you think you might fail, write "fear of failing" on a piece of paper.

- Tape it around one of the rocks.

- Place the rock somewhere where you will look at it often.

- Do this for all of the fears and doubts you carry around with you on a daily basis.

When the day comes that you not only recognize a belief or fear as one that does not serve you but also as one that you do not need any more, you are ready to release it from your "burden backpack." For whatever reason, you are ready to give it no more power in your life.

- Then—and only then—take the label off and put the rock back outside (unless, of course there is a new belief or fear you need to label).

What this exercise does is to make concrete for you the burden of carrying these rocks around with you everyday. There is no pressure to release these doubts and fears until you are ready. But, keep them in front of you so that you can make your choices more consciously every day. Then you can reconnect more easily with the Wisdom within, even if you are not completely ready to listen. You can develop your capacity to have faith in its presence in your life.

We often recognize that there is a greater force than we are, but we lack the faith to give it credit for Wisdom greater than we can comprehend. We instead move to doubt when things don't manifest exactly as we think would be best in the time we expect. If we can't see or understand it, it must be wrong! In one scenario, a successful professional by society's standards, who was used to getting exactly what she wanted, ran into a critical juncture in her life where things didn't appear to be happening as she would have designed. I remember asking her whether she believed that there was a bigger plan than her own. She replied, "Yes." I then asked if she thought there was Wisdom greater that hers that might have a design in mind. She playfully replied, "Yes, but I would rather She or He asked my opinion. I think the plan needs some help!"

Hold a pure intention and hold that it be for the highest good. Then let go of how it should look. It will happen. That's the lesson of faith.

You may find that you are deeply attached to ensuring predictability in various aspects of your life where you want to feel in control. Predictability often provides a false sense of security, the illusion of grounding, and a feeling of control over external circumstances. Predictability requires no faith. You begin to create and live the illusion that you are in charge of life and all its twists and turns. You collude with others to help them feel a sense of predictability in your relationships with them, as well, and block the Wisdom of your heart from showing you what is true.

Conscious living is not about ensuring predictability. Lives inspired by Grace and Wisdom have no need for control. They simply cannot be restrained in that way. As foreign as that may sound to someone who carefully measures every action and response from others, it is true. If the journey to your most inspired Center is one you passionately choose, then the need for control and the willingness to support any illusion of control over Life itself must be surrendered.

Faith frees you to follow your Wisdom, to be true to your Highest Self—unafraid to live that truth in all aspects of your life. You feel free to color outside the lines, dance to your own rhythms, and appreciate your gifts, even if they cause you not to fit with societal, familial, or peer group standards for acceptable behavior. Faith exposes conformity as a major means of control that we collude in reinforcing today. Clarity and courage will indeed support the shattering of any illusions of control and offer in return freedom, truth, joy, and the unleashing of your soul's gifts. Such a choice is supported by listening, with faith, to the Wisdom within—heart, not head. No chatter, just quiet. Faith nurtures your ability to consciously lead your own life—from Wisdom. It also prepares you to nurture new growth.

Before leaving the topic of faith, I would like to offer you a story about the faith involved in sharing the messages in this book with you. The path has taken several twists and turns and definitely required me to be receptive to growth and change.

When I finished my nearly three years of in-dwelling, I set about transcribing relevant portions of my journals to help others on their journey. I got a few error messages in my software—something about a "remote debugger," whatever that is. But I ignored them and continued to enter the data from my journals. I then used the journal entries to structure a three hundred page book, which several friends, colleagues, and clients read—a few read it multiple times. I had chosen each reader carefully for learning styles and writing preferences different from my own and from each other's. Two are editors and three are authors themselves. All gave me gentle suggestions to make the book more reader-friendly. "Add more stories and examples." "Simplify the grammar and word choice."

I made edits—many times. My readers worked with the book again. I sent what I thought was the final version off to a publisher. Not long thereafter, I got my first book rejection. I have to say that the gentleman who called me was wonderful. When he called, I begged him to give me advice and tips on what publishers want. He was most generous. The main point I remember is that my book was "beyond" what his company published. My book was too philosophical. He gently but clearly informed me that to publish the book I had written I needed to be a recognized name—"Oprah" would be a good one! My book simply had a no-name author and no angle that would make it worthy of buyers' attention.

I sent the book off to a friend of a client who has published multiple books. She most kindly forwarded the book to her agent, with encouraging words for me. I also sent it to a third publisher. With no response months later, I contacted a friend and client, who knows quite a lot about both the workshops I have conducted over the years and about marketing in general. She generously agreed to read my manuscript and to provide me feedback. In her beautifully direct and honest style, she told me that the book I had written was wonderful—as a background resource for me to write an engaging book for other readers! She clearly told me that she was not particularly fond of the scholarly voice of the book and missed my "heart voice" that she had experienced in all of my workshops. She told me that she wanted a book that would encourage her to stay with her journey and guide her the whole way through. Oh, and by the way, she expected and could see my artwork playfully dancing on the pages.

I sent a revision of one section of the book to her for review. She told me I simply didn't get it. I needed to write a very different book, one that taught the workshop on being your Best Self, provided explicit exercises, and connected from the heart. Months later, and many people later, I finally heard the message. I reread the original book, took it apart, kept important concepts, and set about writing a very different book. And I thought it was finished. Another year and several more publishing rejections later, I revised the book again. This time I wrote a new introduction and final chapter. After yet another year of insights, I added a chapter, removed another and revised the rest. The process continued. After several years, I had written a very different book—the one you now hold. If I had known what would be required to publish this book from the beginning, I might not have done it. Only through the gradual unfolding and increased clarity about what I wanted to offer those who choose to lead their lives differently, do I now recognize and appreciate the support to stay on path and continue revising.

The opportunities to remember to nurture our unique gardens are many. Clarity, compassion, courage, and faith take different forms in each of our lives at different times. It is up to each of us to choose to be open and connected with the truth in our hearts. When we make the choice to be present in our lives and to listen to what our hearts feel in each moment, the invitation to recognize our attachments to how things are supposed to appear shows up. Until I was finally willing to consider that the messages in my book may need to appear in a radically different way and that I had to essentially throw out the original, I could not see what form would be most helpful to you.

Reestablishing the clarity that getting the messages and tips out there for all who are ready to engage the journey helped me to detach from the time and work I had invested in earlier versions. Compassion tapped me on the shoulder in the process and allowed me to laugh at my Self and the ways I was resisting the path of ease. Faith reminded to let go of how and when you would access the messages in this book and to trust that if what I am bringing to you is important at this time in your life and in our history, the messages will get to you in whatever form works best.

Coach's Tip: Nurture the garden of the heart and Highest Self and weed out the entanglements and distractions of the mind. Stay present and open to opportunities for growth.

Conscious living—by design is the conscious journey back into the human world of Away on the Universal Soul Grid. It is a journey of integration, as you reunite the inner you—Highest Self—with ego-roles and social expectations in new and joyful ways. The following is a brief summary of essential steps and nutrients for *living consciously—by design:*

1. Design your garden for growth

    a. See the relationship for what it is
    b. Weed and prune the garden
         i. Beware of distractions in the garden
        ii. Prepare for goodbyes
    c. Design for new relationships

2. Step into your Grace

    a. Know beauty
    b. Play with life
    c. Trust your intuition
    d. Choose gratitude
    e. Push for clarity and pull opportunity

3. Speak from your heart

    a. Consciously know your intention
    b. Speak your truth
    c. Stay centered when others don't respond from love

4. Lead from Wisdom

    a. Consciously and continuously tend the garden
    b. Essential nutrients
         i. Clarity
        ii. Compassion
       iii. Courage
       iv. Faith

Reflection Checklist (Revisited)

1. Know where you were

2. Know where you are

3. Know where you are headed

Now that you have navigated your way back into the external everyday world, it is again a good time to pause and reflect on where you were, where you are now, and where you are headed. Just as you probably found when you reflected on the journey inward—in-dwelling—to reconnect with your Highest Self at Home, it is much easier to see the order and underlying patterns of your life when you step back from the individual and seemingly disconnected events of every day. With the distance of both space and time, a clearer picture emerges and suddenly the coherence of seemingly unrelated actions and experiences presents itself—without your having to figure anything out!

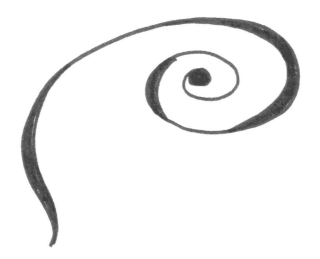

Where you were

Reconnected with your Highest Self and the Wisdom of your heart through the process of in-dwelling at Home, you began to prepare for the journey towards Away—the outer world of human distractions, social norms, and relationships. As you prepared to venture outward, you learned what it takes to move from the solace of your inner sanctuary and the pristine beauty of an undisturbed garden into the noise of human living today. Your first challenge was to be so consciously connected with your heart and its Wisdom that you could stay centered in your truth in the midst of external noise. The preparation you made was to design your life, your garden, in a way that would support living consciously—aware of your choices in every moment. This conscious living—by design involved your grappling with what it means for you to live in your Grace, to be aligned with your truth and essence in every step you take. It was about growing your garden with healthy relationships, according to what supports your Highest Self.

You learned to reconnect with beauty, dance and play with life's rhythms, trust your intuition for guidance, and appreciate what life brings you on your journey. Reestablished in your Grace, you came to understand how you would need to speak from your heart in order to stay in that Grace in the outer world. Staying connected with your own passions, desires, and love while operating among many temptations and distractions to sever the heart connection and give your power to the voices of social convention, fear, and doubt in your head required—and requires—constant vigilance and discipline.

As you became more familiar with the Inner Voice that is uniquely yours, you then became acquainted—or reacquainted—with what it means to listen to your Wisdom in everyday contexts. The choice to follow your Wisdom, empowering your heart to lead the way is the one that beckoned you to nurture your conscious choices with the essential nutrients for growing and maintaining a magnificent garden: clarity, compassion, courage, and faith.

Where you are now*
(*or at least where your Coach thinks you are!)

Today you find your Self poised to more easily integrate your Highest Self—Home—in every aspect of your outer world. You can appreciate the importance of staying consciously attuned to your Inner Wisdom to discern which choices support your purpose and Highest Self. You have experienced the choices that support a path of ease and joy, as well as those that distract you. Conscious living—by design awaits your continuous presence and attention with every step you take on your life's path.

Amidst the clutter and noise of external demands for your attention and time, you are faced with opportunity to stay the course and lead from Wisdom—or to turn away from your Grace and entertain the everyday seduction of busyness and external validation. But this time, you know in your heart the voice of truth and its absolute dedication to supporting your journey. You can ignore this Inner Voice; but you cannot deny its existence—at least not consciously.

Where you are headed

Wherever you choose! The life of joy and ease, contribution and fulfillment—purpose and meaning—awaits your wise and enlightened choices. Others behind and along side you on the journey await your light. The choice to integrate your Highest Self into your everyday life and live into your potential—or not—is entirely up to you. But before you go, there are a few more tips for seeing through the chaos to the underlying coherence of your journey. There are life stage patterns that you may recognize and use to help you be gentler with your Self as you move along the Universal Soul Grid to a more joyful and purpose-filled life. So, for now, relax and watch as the panoramic picture of the path to mastery unfolds before your eyes.

Finding Your Self on the Universal Soul Grid

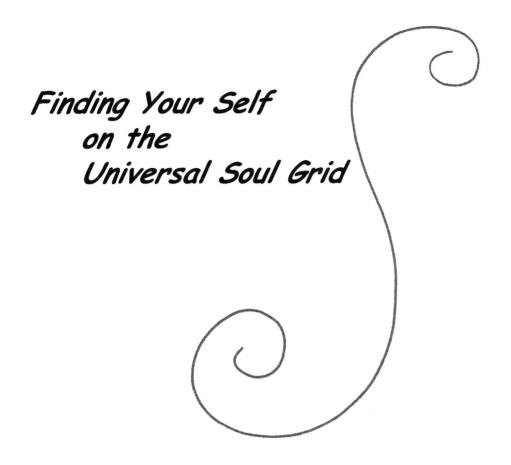

You have ventured inward through the in-dwelling process and at least have a sense of what it takes to live in our everyday world with ease and grace, following the guidance of your heart. Now would be a good time to step back and look at where you are in your life today. Where are you stuck and where are you living with sheer delight? What occupies most of your energy and attention on any given day? Are you finding your energy depleted fighting daily battles at work, home, or in other relationships? Are you finding that you are showing up with a natural Grace that is bringing everything your heart desires—almost before you ask?

Your answers to these questions suggest where you are on the Universal Soul Grid. If you are considered successful by societal measures, or your family and friends' judgments but feel as though something is missing, you may be stuck deep in the Away spiral, needing to reconnect with your true passions and voice. If this is true, know that if you try to hold yourself to the same old measures for success, you will find yourself more tired, less satisfied, and more stuck. You are hanging on for dear life to Away measures for success, when it is time to journey inward towards Home to connect with your heart's inner measures for success. You are being called to test all that has made you successful by others' standards against the levels of joy and fulfillment you currently experience in your life. The next phase of your life requires that you let go of what you have accumulated that you no longer need. It is time to clarify what you want to create and what gifts you want to experience and express. This dynamic of being stuck in Away while called to reconnect at Home occurs over a number of years. It signals a life-stage calling to return to inner truth. How you respond to the prompts to go inward will predict the levels of ease or struggle in your life.

As you assess where you may be stuck or creating resistance, pain, or stress, you may find it helpful to step back and look at a few of the macro-patterns on the soul grid that we humans tend to exhibit at different points in our lives. Perhaps the easiest way to break them down is to consider typical paths that are activated at specific times or ages in your life. The stages offered here are suggested parameters only. Actual ages may vary in your experience. For those of you who are over-achievers, there is no prize for getting there faster! It is far more critical that you be honest with yourself about where you are so that you understand why you feel stuck and what that stuckness is all about.

Remember that the Universal Soul Grid describes a path we walk simultaneously at everyday choice levels and at broader life-stage levels. For example, you may be at a point in your life where you want desperately to work in ways that bring you meaning. You are being prompted to reconnect with your Best Self in order to consciously choose what fulfills your passions and life's purpose. At the same time, your ego identity finds itself trapped in a job that pays the mortgage or health insurance for you and your family. At a micro-level of small daily choices, you may be returning Home to choose those things that make you feel good while toiling at your current job, desperately wanting to quit. You are at Away, bombarded by messages about the "right" thing to do in terms of what your head tells you, while your heart feels heavy. The larger life transition involves smaller decisions everyday that either support or distract you from your Highest Self.

Even as you are aware of the need to clarify whom you choose to be and how you choose to spend your life in the bigger picture, you may find yourself unable to fend off the voices in your head. The back and forth between "shoulds" of your head and emotional truth in your heart may occur continuously in a given day as you choose whether to leave work to see you child's soccer game or sneak in nine holes of golf while looming deadlines demand your attention at work. One way of thinking about what is going on is to consider that you are moving slowly, perhaps imperceptibly, in the macro-pattern of your life stage from Away to Home, while moving constantly at the micro-level between Away and Home. It looks something like this:

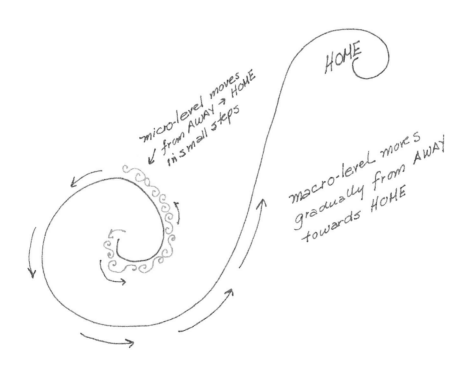

Moving along the soul grid is not a linear process. It is oscillating at the micro-level and iterative at the macro-level, because we are living systems and life doesn't move in straight lines. It can feel messy and chaotic, if you have a need for control (aw, c'mon, not even a little bit?). As you are moving on a macro-path from one end of the soul grid to the other, you are probably going through at least three different stages: experiencing stability, oscillating between old and new, and moving into the unknown (chaos). In the first stage, you try something until it works and you continue to do it until it feels natural and familiar. You get to enjoy it for a little while, it becomes you, and then it is time to change.

In the second stage, if you are unconscious, you resist change, investing every bit of energy in trying to keep things as they were, as you remember them. Even as things are beginning to change around you and you sense a need to change, you try to hold on to the familiar. What is happening is that you are being drawn to move into whatever is next for you on the path of your life. Intuitively you know it is time to move on, but your head registers a form of guilt or anxiety at the prospect of leaving the familiar for the unfamiliar. You are being invited to shed a piece of ego-identity and move into what is more truly you and your voice. This stage is one of oscillation between something new that you don't fully understand or embrace and holding onto what was. It is not unlike completing a grade level of school, being promoted to the next grade level, and wanting to go back to the familiar grade and circumstances in which you felt successful. In a business context, people who are promoted follow the same path. They unconsciously want to continue to do the old work because it is familiar and they know how to succeed at it. If they continue to do so, they never move to new levels of thinking and skills to which they were promoted and the people they manage do not grow or develop either.

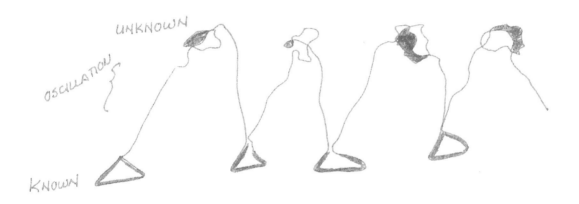

If you keep resisting, you spend a tremendous amount of energy holding on and have little left to feel creative, or to engage what supports your path. You feel caught in transition, neither where you were nor anywhere else. People usually experience this place as a difficult place to be. If you focus on being there, you can create quite a negative tailspin. If you continue to use all your energy holding onto what was, you make the unknown a terrifying prospect and may wear down your immune system as you fight the natural path of growth. If you let go and return Home to your heart to listen to what feels good, to what feels true, you move through both smaller and larger growth transitions easily and reach a new stage of comfort and growth.

The letting go requires both clarity and faith to produce a sense of resolve about detaching and moving on. Once there, you are not particularly worried about how the shifts happen and can be present to notice doors opening for whatever is next in your life. Remember that life simply happens. You are assigning all the meaning. You either make the transition a negative experience of chaos or a positive time of supportive change. Let's consider a specific example of how your response to letting go can either create fear and suffering or ease in moving on with your life.

If you are a parent of adolescents and your identity comes from being needed by your children to guide them, you may find yourself challenged between holding onto what the relationship used to be and discovering what is needed now, for both you and your young adults. For both your children's sakes and your own life, you are being invited to redefine your relationship with your children. They no longer need you to tie their shoes, yet you may not be ready to let go because who you have become in life has been defined by how you parent your children. When your children reach a stage where they understand right from wrong and are moving into taking accountability for their own choices, you are also given the opportunity to grow into what is next in your life—so that everybody can grow. You are being asked to rethink your ways of helping your children, and to let go of actions and roles that have become your identity.

Some parents are not ready to engage their own passions beyond being Mom or Dad, often because they shut those other passions down to be parents. This is precisely the point where many parents unconsciously resist their own journey inward, creating more dependent relationships with their children. In trying to be involved in aspects of their children's lives when it is time for the children to make their own choices, these parents unwittingly slow the child's journey. Holding on out of fear is a distraction, and you know it by the levels of resistance and pain that accompany your choices. If you look more closely, you will find that you are being prodded internally to reconnect with your passions, to step into the next phase of your life. If you refuse to let go because you do not know what that next phase is, you can get stuck and entwined in head messages, unable to use the space that children used to fill to clarify your own passions and desires. Look carefully at any resistance you may be getting from your children who are being pulled towards what is next in their lives. Consider reframing that resistance as a signal to you to step back, for both your children's sake and yours, to regain perspective.

It is your opportunity to let go, develop the capacity to listen to your heart, and welcome what is next on your path. When you do, the transition inward is much easier and you shift from being stuck to feeling liberated. You are being asked to release the ego-identity you learned when you moved from Home to Away, mastering what it takes to parent successfully in our society. You are being asked to look more closely at who you have become and choose what to keep and what to discard, based on what you love and what fills you, for the next phase of your life.

There is nothing to figure out or engineer. What supports your next step is paying attention to what drains you and what energizes you in every conversation, every relationship, and every situation. Pay attention. Tell the truth. Give your Self permission to admit that you do not know what you really want in your heart. Holding on is resisting what is changing and resistance creates stress. What is asked is that you let go, face your fears of being still, and hear your heart's truth.

All the old messages about selfishness and responsibility play in your head as you discern between head and heart. Daily decisions tempt you back to Away and the identity you built in the external world of your past, even as your life stage is calling you Home to reconnect with your Highest Self. The stages and stuckness are predictable. By recognizing the basic patterns of your particular life-stage, you can know that you are not alone, release the fear, and move more easily into what awaits your voice and gifts. Let's look more closely at a few patterns.

Life-stage patterns

We can consider the general momentum for the first two decades of life to be outward. We start at Home, unconscious of who we are. Little children are quite happy to follow their hearts without question or fear of consequence. They know what they want in the present moment and usually make those desires known. As children learn to play with other children and interact in social settings, they also learn what behaviors are considered acceptable. They begin to discover what is rewarded, what gets them approval, love, or acceptance. They unconsciously learn to listen more to these external messages than to the inner calls of their hearts, especially once they enter school. The journey outward from Home and the heart's clear wisdom, towards Away and the external messages of authority, society and media, is one that is occurring during the child's formative years. It is an unconscious process of accumulating labels and ego-identity, relationships, and things.

If we fast-forward to young adults in their twenties, the focus is still on movement towards Away, towards achieving success according to societal or peer group standards. They have, by this time, learned to tell themselves that these external standards and measures matter to them. They have accepted external measures of success as their own. The first thirty plus years of life focus outward on fitting into external rules and roles. This focus outward is accompanied by a zest for acquiring things and relationships. The twenties are a time of great learning—about relationships, intimacy, setting up home, establishing a career, succeeding in a variety of work and social environments, and so on. It is a time of great energy—needing less sleep and compartmentalizing activities in order to do more of everything that is out there to be experienced.

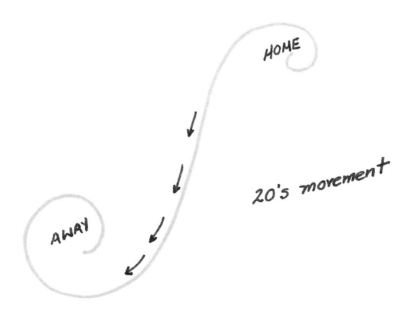

Somewhere in the early to mid-thirties, we begin to sense a call to mastery. It often comes knocking in the vague awareness of feeling scattered and wanting to be really good at something. There is sometimes a sense of feeling like an imposter, especially if you are successful by society's measures and not internally convinced of your unique strengths. Not quite sure what it is that makes you an expert in your chosen field, you worry that if someone else looks too deeply, there might be nothing there to justify your success. The call to mastery or discipline helps create a need to focus attention and energy on specific chosen areas—work, home, hobby, or some area of study that is associated with a sense of personal accomplishment, self-worth, or identity. It is the ego-identity that is rewarded by being better at something than other people are. Being known as the star buys us membership in the eyes of those whose approval we seek. The relevant portion of the soul grid journey that is active during this stage is the lower loop, the inner rings of the Away spiral. It is a time of going deeper to levels of mastery, after the twenties of experiencing broadly.

The thirties signal a time for mastery of human expectations to belong, contribute, to feel recognized and worthy—all measured by external judgments and standards of Away. The generalist at work has been paying attention to what she or he is rewarded for and works at to become the best. The educator develops and refines a practice that is his or her own and gets results that others recognize. The company employee develops even more powerful connections with a specific "known for" that others value. The artist hones technique and personal style. All develop what might be thought of as a brand identity—something that marks each one by her or his unique value in a crowded market or field. It is a time of great productivity and achievement, as measured by titles, positions, relationships, possessions, and financial gain.

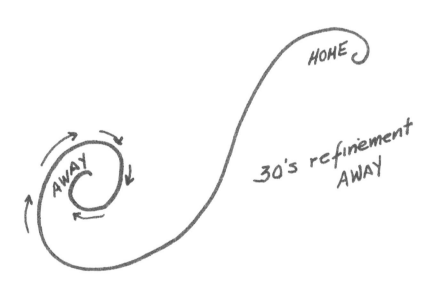

As you develop success Away, a slight shift begins to take place. It often takes the form of a vague sense of emptiness in the late thirties to a more conscious awareness of trying to do too much in the early forties. Often there is a vague questioning of why—after having achieved success in what you set out to do—you feel empty or tired. There is a sense of spending a lot of energy and feeling as though you are on a hamster's wheel, running faster and never really feeling complete or satisfied. If you are at work, you are thinking about home. If you are at home, you are checking e-mail. You never experience the fulfillment of being completely present in either place. The titles, if you are honest, don't feel as shiny or impressive as they once did or as you had expected they would. The things you have acquired may bring a smile, but rarely sustained joy.

What is happening at this point is the gentle nudge inward towards Home. You have been acquiring skills and experiences that prepare you for more fundamental contributions later in life, but you have no conscious measures for their ultimate value. They are measured today in terms of things acquired. Titles that used to raise you up now wear you down. Big homes require more resources. Impressive jobs rob you of relaxation and celebrating simple everyday miracles. The acquisitions have become weights on your journey. It is time to shift from decades of accumulation to a period of more conscious reflection. It is time to sift through all you are carrying with you on this journey called life to determine what still nourishes the best in you and what simply wears you down. You are being prompted to shift from decades of unconscious accumulation to consciously taking inventory of who you have become. It is time to release, to let go of all that does not serve you on your path.

Many of us will fight this urge to look closely at who we have become and what our lives are about because we are not accustomed to looking at our lives so consciously. It feels foreign—and to some, scary. We have spent approximately forty years of our lives mastering this game of what it means to be successful in human terms, rarely questioning why we are choosing what we do or alternatively telling ourselves that we have no choice if what we want is "x." The early forties herald a major shift in becoming more conscious of our experiences, more discerning, and more inwardly focused in order to prepare for our true work in the world. It is time to shift from an outward focus of external measures and distractions from our heart's voice to the inner Wisdom that guides our paths. This is the journey from Away towards Home. It is precisely the stage illustrated in the earlier example of the parents of adolescents who grapple with releasing roles that no longer serve them or their children, yet provide a familiar identity.

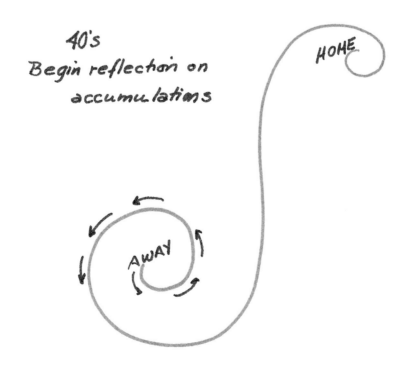

It is a time when head and heart are often at odds. You unconsciously push to hold onto old roles and measures of productivity, while the voice of your heart pushes for joy, ease, and meaning. In the early forties—you begin to monitor what you are getting for what you invest in relationships with family, friends, work, and community. During this time the emotional and physical energy invested versus rewards returned to you begins to get your attention. It is a time of recalibrating and honestly looking at what gives you meaning, brings joy, and is worthy of your energy and life force.

An interesting thing begins to occur at this point, as you are being prompted to shift your attention inward. You notice that the luster disappears from the shiny titles and possessions. Something feels uneasy. For some people the vague sense of emptiness or feeling little or no joy in who they have become or how they are investing their energy is terrifying. This group sets about pushing harder to accumulate things and tangible measures of worth, desperately seeking to hold onto the identity they have built. Some develop a singular focus on getting promoted or attaining assignments that continue to focus their energy outward, allowing them to deny any inner awareness of the emptiness that they experience. Others seek younger partners or flashy toys in efforts to medicate themselves from the strange pressure to look inward.

This particular response can be especially painful—think mid-life crisis—because holding onto what was is a direct resistance to life's calling on the soul grid to go inward. At a time when we are prompted to clarify who we want to be and what we want our lives to be about, some of us resist looking with all the energy we can muster—many to the point of physical illness and emotional turmoil. From Botox to antidepressants and thyroid medications, we use whatever allows us to deny the call inward, to avoid engaging in-dwelling in order to find our unique voice and truth.

One reason so many of us medicate ourselves from feeling the call inward is the painful awareness that we have no idea what we want, other than some vague notion of inner peace, satisfaction, or passion. All of those years of powering through life, proving your worth in human terms, and attaining externally-validated milestones begin to feel empty or meaningless when you realize that you have no idea what your passions and desires are anymore. They have been supplanted by the wants, needs, and shoulds of the voices in your head. Continuing to listen to the voices in your head tell you that you have the perfect life or at least a secure job, home, or other tangible assets requires you to depress the voice in your heart, as it tries to tell you that something is missing, that you want something more or different.

The response of some people at this point is to shut down their feelings and emotions in any way they can. Avoidance and denial may find their expression in doing too much of anything to avoid stillness or being alone with feelings and doubts. Becoming stuck and unable to do anything is another response. Away is familiar and you are being called Home. Will you resist and create painful transitions by oscillating between what no longer fulfills you and what you want to create with your precious life? Or will you let go and tumble gently into the unfamiliar, trusting that you will discover and strengthen your resolve to live from your Highest Self, stepping into the uniqueness that is you?

If you listen to that sense of emptiness and do not allow the vagueness of the initial prompts to go inward to scare you, you come to a point of honesty where you question what experiences you want from your life. Some people begin to focus on mortality and legacy, others on wanting to direct their energy in more satisfying ways. Where you are on the soul grid is on the bottom loop Away, sensing a need or desire to reconnect with what you like about yourself, who you really are when you strip away the roles you play to impress others. You are being prompted to identify what brings you inner peace and joy.

It is a time when you naturally want to conserve your energy, even if you do not know why. You are drawn to find quiet time, space to just be. Vaguely disturbed by outside demands on your time you begin to crave "me time." The call inward beckons in the early forties, if not before. If you begin to create that space for in-dwelling, you find yourself beginning to let go of some of your accumulations, including relationships where you are doing all the work and getting less than what you really want in return. You begin to notice the voices in your head that have told you to be thankful for what you have and to stop questioning. You start to notice how much energy it takes to defy your heart and give power to these head voices that no longer ring true.

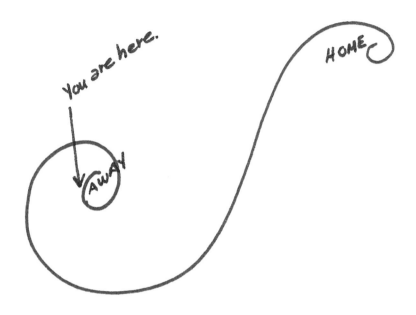

As you begin to create the space to pay attention to physical symptoms of energy drain and general health, you move into consciously choosing to be more aware of what brings you joy, what fills you up. This process continues into the late forties and early fifties when the push for meaning accelerates. You look more carefully at work and relationships that you may have been willing to sustain in your youth that just don't feel worth the effort anymore. Your patience for activity that does not fulfill you or give you a sense of purpose and meaningful contribution drops drastically. It is a time of simplifying and wanting to only invest your time and energy in what you consider essential. Some find themselves wanting to redecorate their homes more simply, often cleaning closets of accumulated things they no longer want. It is about perfecting the inward calling to spend time with your Highest Self. The focus on spending your time and energy well grows more prominent in your daily activities.

In the fifties the journey towards Home continues, as you more consciously choose who you will be, what you like about your Self and your life, and where you will spend your talents and energies. You move away from the shoulds and more honestly question what you want. The value for integrity increases, as does the prominence of legacy. In the fifties, many things are turned upside down, as what you had been told and told your Self was important and mattered a great deal becomes less important. Little everyday things that you used to think of as unimportant—making time to share a cup of tea with a friend or listening intently to a child's story—become more important. It is a time of shifting priorities. And as with the forties, if you resist the invitation to listen to your Inner Wisdom, you will find ample opportunities to entertain the voices in your head, living your life for the morsels of approval and validation doled out by others.

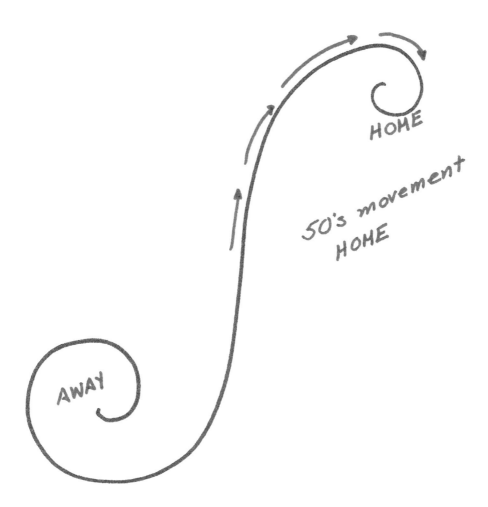

If you follow the natural momentum inward, towards Home, without resistance, you learn to recognize the costs of trying to be someone or something different from your Highest Self. You build the clarity, and what some would call courage, to know how to choose whatever or whoever supports your living in the joy of the present. When you are fully aware of the ease of traveling lightly, without the shoulds and with the voice of Inner Wisdom guiding your choices, you are also beginning to shift momentum outward towards Away *more consciously.* This time you are appearing outwardly different to other people.

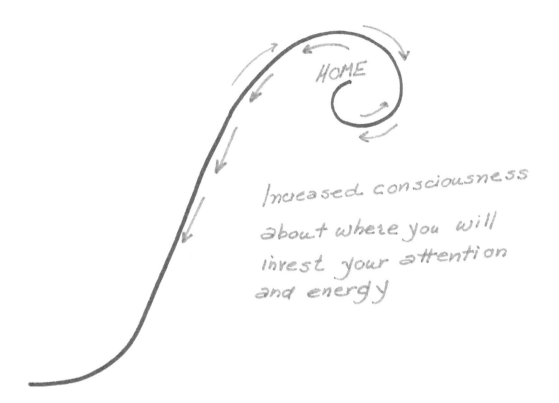

HOME

Increased consciousness about where you will invest your attention and energy

Somewhere between your mid- fifties and early sixties, you carefully consider every idea, relationship, or activity as an invitation, rather than an obligation, for you to invest the energy of who you are and what you want to bring to life.   In this context, saying "no" is absolutely essential and something you do with clarity. You also learn to do it without guilt or apology, as the call to serve the best in you drives your choices.

The clarity portion of stepping fully into your Grace will take the next decade or so, as you navigate the world of Away without losing touch with the conscious Highest Self from Home. The path of integration takes over the earlier years of learned compartmentalization, as you make your decisions from a conscious Center. You seek out situations that celebrate who you are, not ones that ask you to change to fit in. You understand that the old attempts to balance life were mirages. Life is not to be balanced. It is to be lived from the core of your Best Self in every relationship and situation. You are more able to live *in* the world without being *of* it—blissfully detached from external measures of your success as a human being. You find yourself deeply connected with the truth of your heart and the Wisdom of your intuition, or Inner Voice. Instead of others' judgments, it is your own truth and clear intention that guide your choices every day. You are choosing to withdraw your energy from relationships and parts of your life that no longer inspire or fulfill you. They no longer fit who you are becoming.

In the latter third of life—mid sixties through nineties—you do what brings you joy. To whatever brings you meaning, you lend the voice of your Highest Self in ways that are free, full, and fulfilling. You are living consciously Away, continuing to integrate your Highest Self in every relationship and situation in which you engage. Everyone you touch stands to benefit from you living into your purpose—unabashedly. Everything you have done and learned has prepared you to integrate your Best Self in each step of your journey. You carry Home in conscious decisions Away. When seduced by the clamor of the outside world, you step back to reconnect with the core of you. The pressure to succeed by society's measures decreases in later years as elders take their place as wise advisors—simply by being true to the best and highest in themselves.

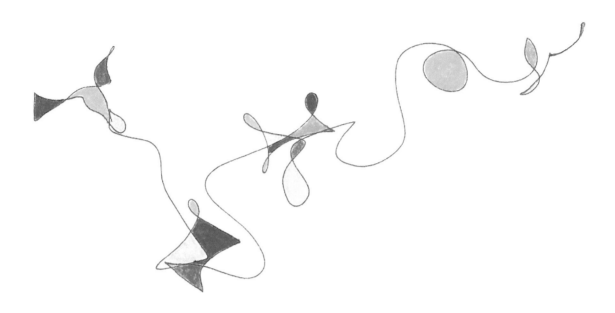

If you look around our world today, it will be fairly clear to you that not everyone follows the calls of the Universal Soul Grid inward or outward at the points suggested here. Some will deliberately seek the counsel of friends and family to reinforce old patterns, regain a sense of normalcy, and hang onto the past for dear life, since moving forward means letting go and allowing life to unfold. Instead of expanding into their Highest Selves, they contract and shrink from their own brilliance. A pattern of more difficult transitions in life often follows these people. They oscillate between listening to their hearts and embracing the unknown, and listening to the fearful voices in their heads, becoming paralyzed and stuck in old patterns. They are essentially hanging onto one trapeze while longing to have the courage to grab onto the one life is throwing them. By refusing to let go of the past and ego-identity, they just keep swinging and telling themselves all sorts of wonderful things to keep themselves from grabbing the new ring. Sound familiar?

What does this mean for you?

The timelines outlined here are suggested guidelines for recognizing paths to joy and ease. If you overlay your particular journey on the Soul Grid, you will likely find the places where you have chosen resistance and stress over consciously easing into the fullest expression of your Highest Self. The good news is that you can shift at any point to get back on your path. Skip the self-critical judgments. Welcome any awareness of the desire to create what you want in your life, the desire to more fully express the very best in you. Focus your attention on the person you consciously choose to be and listen carefully for the prompts that life offers you. Create graceful opportunities to get right back on path—and do it!

Remember that the soul grid movement from and to Away is more organic and iterative than linear. What this means is that you may feel as though you sometimes take two steps forward and one back. If you step back, you may be able to see that you are reconnecting with who you are in small daily decisions even as you move Away in bigger life patterns. The macro-level movements we often recognize as transitions. We tend to experience these transitions as more gradual movement, as we navigate towards one end of the Universal Soul Grid or the other. Keep in mind that daily choices that cause you to either touch base with Home or Away while moving in the opposite direction are part of the process of becoming more conscious. And becoming more conscious is what prepares you to create a life of joy and ease.

As you move through transitions in one direction or the other, you will repeat a core pattern called the mastery path. You may engage it consciously or unconsciously. Regardless of what part of the journey you are on, this basic pattern connects seemingly disparate events and situations. If you consciously recognize its existence, you have the opportunity to create even more ease in your journey because what might have appeared random takes on new meaning. And it can be quite exciting!

Path to

Mastery

The extraordinary beauty and light that emanate from one who is in her or his Grace is undeniable. There is no tempering or restraint to fit with social convention. There is no spin on the message to appeal to a given audience. Grace is not about doing. It is purely about being. The stillness and peace that accompany vibrant boldness express all that is natural and true within your soul. You hunger to know your own greatness, to live in your Grace. You may also be hesitant to face the unknown.

All the lessons of in-dwelling lead to a life of Grace. You may want repeatable steps—a formula—for how you "do" or "get" Grace. They don't exist. The only steps are the ones you take to live into your truth. The path to stillness, silence, and presence allows you to boldly plumb the depths of your soul to become consciously aware of what is true for you. Living in Grace means nourishing what moves in you, saying "yes" to heart's callings. It is the opposite of medicating to avoid feeling in order to push through the next stage of something or a relationship's challenge. Life isn't something to "get through." Recognize the tendency to reward your Self with eating, drinking, or spending money for having gotten through something. These are medications to anesthetize your Self from the awareness of not being fully present in your life. Such medications are not the path to ease or graceful living. They are only a distraction, a desperate attempt by the mind to help you override the truth in your heart.

If you are waiting for proof that the courageous step you need to take will work out, you are not on path. Let go already! Get quiet. Trust your heart. Be gentle with your Self. Compassion will go a lot farther in opening your heart than harsh judgment. Some people want to plan everything to make sure there are no surprises. When you are in your Grace, you recognize that planning may need to look very different from the way many individuals and organizations plan today. Instead of setting a goal, laying out all of the steps, and rushing quickly to action focused only on the steps you had planned, remember the alternative approach is to *push for clarity at the center and pull the support you want from opportunities that you observe.*

Notice that in this approach, you do not get attached to any specific steps, which means that you can receive direction when it appears. Recognize that the approach to ease and grace does not support your need for control. If you must plan, consider that it is less about planning the actual steps and more about creating the clarity to be able to consciously choose what serves your intention. It is about preparing the soil. It requires that you be fully present in your heart.

When you get some distance from the choices that you have been consciously making to follow your heart, you will notice that the universe supports a gradual mastery process. You first practice making decisions that support your path in relationships that are relatively low risk—meaning that you are less afraid of being rejected or losing that particular relationship if things don't work out as you imagined they would. Initially the circumstances may present themselves for you to practice a new behavior that serves your path—such as taking a stand for something you want or disagreeing with someone whose approval you want—in the check-out line at the store or on a train with people you don't know. It is relatively safe for you to risk rejection or disapproval in these contexts because these people are not a critical part of your emotional support system.

Typically, the path to mastery involves facing the distraction that takes you from your path in a setting or with individuals who are not close to your heart or financial security. It is safer for you to practice where you feel anonymous. As you continue to practice making choices that align with your heart's Wisdom, you will find that you are given opportunities with people you know, perhaps acquaintances at your place of worship or a community organization. You will practice the same behaviors—maybe learning to say "no" or speak your own truth—in increasingly familiar and more intimate settings. Again, your clarity will either keep you on path or be insufficient to counteract the noise and unconscious pressure to give in to immediate comfort and predictable patterns of your ego-identity.

For example, you may be able to accept someone's offer for you to cut in line at the grocery store when you have only one item, but have difficulty accepting an offer to have a neighbor drive your children because your head tells you that it is your responsibility to drive them. Whatever the rules in your head for being a "good neighbor" or "responsible parent," if you listen to and follow these rules, you allow your ego-role identity to distract you from your path. Your lack of clarity about whatever you are learn-ing to support in your life—perhaps taking a stand for health or healthy boundaries in what you agree to do—is contributing to your decisions to follow your distractions rather than creating new boundaries that support your Highest Self.

Even if you have been standing strong against conventional wisdom, in support of your own journey, there will come points where you may cave to distractions. When you do, you are likely to do it often enough that you fall into an old pattern. What typically happens to get your attention again is that the heat is turned up. Several people close to you—whether at work, at home, or both—challenge you to remember who you are at your Center. You may find that you feel overwhelmed and lost for a while. Remember not to judge your Self harshly. Simply stop. Look carefully at what is. Create quiet to clarify what you consciously choose in the situation and get back on the journey! Remember—graceful exits and graceful entries—no matter how many times. Here is a concrete example to illustrate:

Early in my own journey, I made the choice not to use e-mail. This was a conscious choice. As a socio-linguist, I derive more than half the data I use to help clients from hearing the client's voice. I believed that fostering e-mail connections would increase my workload and decrease my effectiveness significantly. I also did not want to be tethered to technology. As a frequent flier, I would have needed either to carry a computer with me or to work weekends to answer e-mails received during the week—neither of which I chose to do. I made my choice not to play by conventional rules. Some of the early reactions to my decision surprised me.

A former colleague that I met at a reunion accused me of being arrogant because I refused to be available to him in the manner—e-mail—and at the times when it was most convenient for him to contact me. The potential distraction for me was the accusation of being arrogant. I could not understand why my decision would be seen as arrogant and I did not want to be seen this way. However, on conscious reflection, I stayed with my decision—despite conventional pressures to change it. I released any need to address how he was judging me.

The dilemma continued as potential new clients informed me that their preferred way of communicating was e-mail. Considering the potential cost to the business of losing such clients, I weighed again the decision not to be accessible by e-mail. I was already accessible by cell phone and committed to returning client calls within a day or two. I continued to address each individual prospective client in turn. Each one seemed flabbergasted that anyone could even operate in today's business world without e-mail, not to mention a PDA for immediate response needs! When I listened very carefully to potential clients' responses—and I was up front with them right from the beginning—most reluctantly admitted they wished they could do the same.

As I continued with this decision, some of my current clients began to contact my business partner, who is accessible through e-mail, to contact me or to forward written documents to me. I made a conscious pact with my business partner that my refusal to use e-mail with clients would not increase her workload. I notified any client who tried to contact me through her that that option was not available and that she would not be forwarding any messages she received for me through e-mail.

I recognize that my decision causes inconvenience for people who are used to operating primarily through e-mail. I am prepared to be out of the loop or not a part of relationships that depend on e-mail for their sustainability. However, I am clear—at least for today—that being available to clients and friends via e-mail does not serve my Best Self. If the cost is clients who refuse to do business with someone who will not work weekends, or commit to checking e-mail when I get up in the morning and before going to bed at night, I am prepared to assume that cost, walk away from that business, and find other ways to generate income.

The specific topic of using e-mail is not the point here. The point is that whatever your path, you will make decisions that pit your clarity against conventional wisdom and the preferences of other people. If you are not clear about your intention, it will be difficult for you to stand firmly when challenged. This is not about becoming rigid in a decision made at one point in your life. In fact, the path to mastery is exactly the opposite. It requires that once you make a decision, you continue to ask, each time you are faced with a choice that challenges what you believe to be your truth, what decision is true for you *in that moment*. When conditions change, you may choose to change your position.

If you should cave to the distractions of your head at any point on your journey, recognize that when you come back to your path, you will need to pick it up where you left off, if you want to create the life of joy that is yours to have. Once you have practiced standing for your truth and following your Wisdom in "safer" contexts, you will continue to clarify your intention by choosing your truth in more intimate contexts.

Risking the rejection of family, close friends, employer, spouse, or partner challenges you to remember that your ultimate soul mate is your Highest Self and that your true security in life is neither financial nor emotional. It is the integrity of your life—your wholeness. When you carry that clarity within you, you walk your path with ease and joy—detached from emotional ties to how the journey looks. Instead you are most deeply connected to your Inner Wisdom, your heart's truth.

If your particular path is related to being able to take a stand for what you believe in a way that feels true to you, then you might be attracting—consciously or unconsciously—opportunities to practice standing up for your Self. Perhaps you dislike conflict and continually find yourself in environments with argumentative people. Until you begin to change your response to those people, you will continue to attract the situations that you need to master if you want to step into your life's potential. Once you have mastered your new skills with people you are prepared to disappoint, or whose approval you decide you don't need, you will begin to attract similar behaviors and situations with people closer to you—until you don't need the practice anymore.

Coach's Tip: If you pay attention to what you are attracting in your life—frustration or joy, people who bring out the best in you or those around whom you shut down—you can see through the disparate events to the more fundamental choice that you need to make to follow your Wisdom.

At some point, assuming you are staying present and paying attention, you will notice the pattern of what you are attracting and understand why. From that point on, your clear intention about the kind of person you want to be in a relationship and the kind of relationship that is worth your life force becomes a magnet for these kinds of relationships. Your choices become clearer and your resolve stronger to remove the blocks or distractions from your path. You will also discover that major transition points in your life are especially helpful in highlighting what you are attracting and what needs to change.

The more consciously you live your life, and more present you are, the easier it is to see the patterns in seemingly disparate or chaotic events. You may find that someone directs you to a book. You do nothing about it. Days or weeks later, you run across an article naming the same book. If you still don't do anything about it, you may get a third reference. Pay attention to the message and to your body or emotional response. Watch the pattern reveal itself to you. A dear and wise friend, on losing her battle to cancer once told me, "Don't wait for the neon." The signs are on your path every day. They only get more dramatic and louder when you don't pay attention.

Your level of resistance to hearing the invitation to move the roadblocks and get on your own path of ease and purpose is directly related to the degree of difficulty in your life. The path itself does not need to be as hard as we often make it. Unconscious attachments get in the way. Pay attention to what you are attracting in your life and how you are responding to what you attract to understand how far off your design for conscious living you really are.

Coach's Tip: Release resistance and make faith your partner in greeting the unknown on the journey to live consciously.

Get back on the path and play. Dance with Life again. When you choose bold action to support heart's desire and express your truth, you create a field of unrestricted movement for your Self. You find resources that have eluded you in the past. The world feels as if it stands before you awaiting your call. Everything you try seems to work with ease. When you trust your heart, live your purpose, and lead from Wisdom, your path unfolds before you.

> *Bet the farm...The real game awaits those who play from and with heart. Choose your bold play with a sense of openness, playfulness, curiosity...When you bring your focus in line with your energy and form, you win...What you hold dear manifests. Just play with heart.*

The full color and magnificence of the garden that is your Highest Self awaits your full expression.

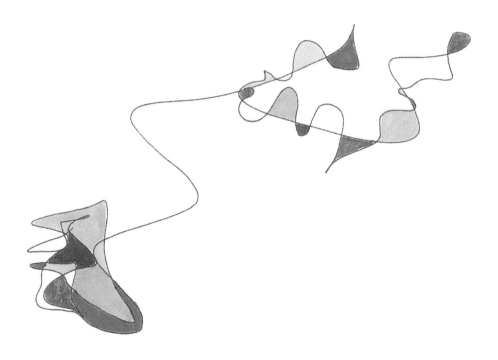

The art of Being is knowing
in every cell of our bodies
the texture and brilliance of our essential nature
and
expressing it through our unique gifts.

The ultimate masterpiece begins with a journey inward
to the depths of silence,
beyond
the reaches of the mind's constructs,
ego's need to maintain the status quo by hiding the unconscious
from our conscious awareness,

to a place
where the clarity of our Self shines brilliantly, in a spectacular burst of
color and light.

And as we shine our light on our Truths,
we individually and collectively become
Co-Creators of a conscious existence
Lived in the Present
Loved for its Splendor
and
shared in every dimension of our
Individual and Collective
Being

Knowing all the while
that we are the Designers and the Design
of a new way of Being
in Relationship with our Selves
and
Each Other
on the planet

Let go of how much time and energy you have invested in what you have and in who you are today. If you hold on to the familiar, you won't have a free hand to embrace the new. What would you need to fully embrace the extraordinary beauty of your garden, to give your gifts and passions their fullest expression in your life?

It is said that if you catch a fly and put a lid on the jar with holes for air, the fly will learn the limitations of its space. At a later point in time, you can take the cap off the jar and the fly will not leave—because it does not know that it can. Raising your awareness about ways that you make choices that unconsciously limit your Self from your magnificence is the work of in-dwelling. The process simply cannot be understood by the rational mind in other than a very limited way until you actually experience the spaciousness of your Highest Self directly. You have been taught to constrain your Self from the time you were a child. The gift of in-dwelling is not only the vibrancy and peace it brings to life; it is also the promise of continuous support through a deep connection with the Wisdom of your heart. Conscious living is not a part time job. The promise of a purposeful and joy-filled life that supports your Highest Self exists in every choice of every moment.

The journey inward is an invitation to meet the truth of your Self deep within your soul. The gift you give to your Self and the people you touch on your journey outward is the very best of who you are, and the pure Wisdom that supports the highest in all of us. You are invited to live a life of Grace, recognizing your own path, and ensuring that the decisions you make and the energy you invest in every relationship support your Highest Self.

> *In choosing to follow your heart's wisdom, you leave behind whispers of fear and imposed barriers to splendid growth. Choose Light and live Wisdom. Create the path for others to follow as they select spiritual awakening. Now.*

It is about choosing who you will be in every moment of every day. It is about answering the call to become your Highest Self in ways that invite everyone you touch to do the same.

It is about creating the experiences of our wildest imaginings for all of us on this planet, from every walk of life, to be free to choose consciously how we will contribute. It is about human and social potential.

It is about being. The choice is each of ours to make. We get to make it every day. And if we get lost for a while, we are welcomed back on the path whenever we are ready, fully embraced and supported in consciously creating our world.

It is about…

Essence

In apparent chaos, there is order
  There is Divine Wisdom, and knowing that passes all understanding
Abiding Faith carries through the darkness caused by amnesia
  A forgetting of the ultimate Wisdom
That we are all connected in our Essence
  One as co-creators and created
Born to remember, reunite the apparently separate worlds
  Through a deep, resounding Grace
Permeating our individual and collective consciousness
  Inviting nothing less than all of us
To Be—nothing less than each of us is
Complete and whole and
  One with all of Creation

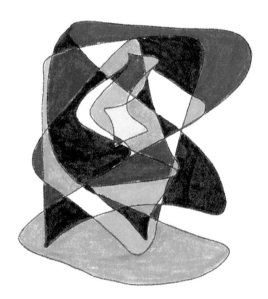

The journey of ***humans being*** beckons.

Imagine who you will be…

Imagine what all of us will create together as **humans being**…consciously

    one choice at a time,

        one person at a time,

            one world at a time.

Ready?

        Your turn.

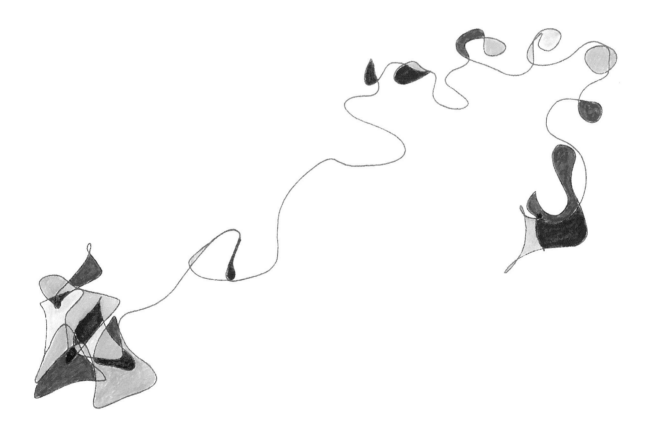

Glossary

AWAY The place on the Soul Grid that represents the outermost external focus. It is the place of highest connection with what it means to be human and to be accepted by human standards.

AWAY-HOME The phase on the Universal Soul Grid that represents a time of releasing or shedding the parts of life that no longer serve your Highest Self. It signals a contraction phase that focuses inward.

BEST SELF See Highest Self.

DISTRACTION Refers to a force that is designed to help the Soul be aware of the qualities it came to experience. Each person has a primary means of distraction that tempts one to abandon life's purpose in favor of what appears to be an easier path.

EGO-IDENTITY The identity accumulated through outward focus. It comprises the qualities one adopts from what others have said about him or her. It is an unconsciously developed human identity.

ESSENCE The purest form of who you are at your core—your qualities and gifts.

HEART'S DESIRE An expression of the deepest passions and truth within your heart. As used in this book, heart's desire serves Highest Self and life purpose.

HIGHEST SELF Who you are at your core; the very best in qualities that uniquely map to your truth. Highest Self is the opposite of ego-identity.

HOME That place on the Universal Soul Grid that houses Highest Self and Divine truth.

HOME-AWAY Refers to the expansion and outer-focused phase of the Universal Soul Grid. When describing an unconscious earlier stage in life, it is an accumulation phase associated with ego-identity.

IN-DWELLING   Process of focusing your intensity inward to plumb the depths of your heart and soul; means to accessing Highest Self.

INNER VOICE   The voice of truth and Wisdom housed within each person's heart. It is accessed through in-dwelling.

INTUITION   A way of knowing that is whole, immediate, and inspired. It is the opposite of rational processes in that it cannot be broken down into its component parts. It is heard through Inner Voice when you have no ties to what message it is sending. Often referred to as "gut sense."

SOUL GRID   Refers to an invisible track that humans travel throughout a lifetime. The Universal Soul Grid describes the pathway that is true for all humans. It is represented by a spiral "S." Individual soul grids describe the unique patterns of each person relative to individual distraction and life purpose.

SPACIOUSNESS   The condition of expanding into your full Self without limitation; fullest expression of Highest Self.

Table of Exercises

End Notes

1. Andreas, Brian. *Hearing Voices. StoryPeople*, 1998. Reprinted with permission of Brian Andreas.
2. Hawkins, David. *Power versus Force: The Hidden Determinants of Human Behavior.* Hay House, 1995.
3. Ganim, Barbara and Susan Fox. *Visual Journaling: Going Deeper than Words.* The Theosophical Publishing House, Quest Edition, 1999.
4. Underwood, Paula. Workshop presentation, 2000.
5. Rumi. *The Essential Rumi: Expanded Edition* translated by Coleman Barks, HarperCollins Publishers, 2004. Reprinted with permission of Coleman Barks.
6. Williamson, Marianne. *A Return to Love: Reflections on the Principles of A Course in Miracles,* HarperCollins Publishers, 1992. Chapter 7, p. 190-191.

About the Author

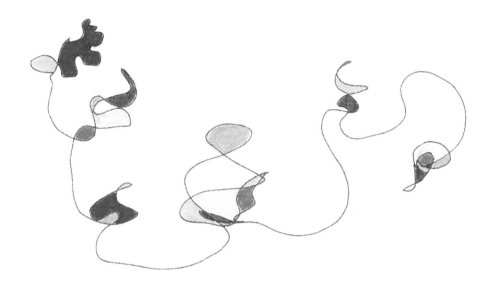

Lou Ann Daly, Ph.D. is a sociolinguist who approaches life with a sense of discovery and an insatiable love of learning and beauty. She delights in the arts, flourishes in helping people step into their potential and unique gifts, and is a natural teacher. She has held a variety of leadership positions in academic, business, and consulting environments. In addition to serving as a life and career coach to executives, Lou Ann has delivered keynote addresses and workshops to clients from countries around the world.

With a designer's sensibilities and an artist's soul, Lou Ann co-founded O! LAD, Organization for Life Architecture and Design, Inc, an organization dedicated to raising emotional health and consciousness in this world, by helping individuals and organizations to clarify their essential nature and purpose, and to design ways to live into their gifts and unique voice with joy and ease. She can most often be found laughing with clients, family, and friends along the rocks and beaches of Maine and Massachusetts.